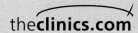

theclinics.com

ULTRASOUND CLINICS

Obstetric Ultrasound

Guest Editor

DEBORAH LEVINE, MD

Gynecologic Ultrasound

Guest Editor

SHEILA SHETH, MD

April 2007 • Volume 2 • Number 2

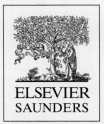

ELSEVIER
SAUNDERS

An imprint of Elsevier, Inc
PHILADELPHIA LONDON TORONTO MONTREAL SYDNEY TOKYO

W.B. SAUNDERS COMPANY
A Division of Elsevier Inc.

1600 John F. Kennedy Boulevard ● Suite 1800 ● Philadelphia, Pennsylvania 19103-2899

http://www.theclinics.com

ULTRASOUND CLINICS Volume 2, Number 2
April 2007 ISSN 1556-858X, ISBN-13: 978-1-4160-5130-5, ISBN-10: 1-4160-5130-9

Editor: Barton Dudlick

Reprints: For copies of 100 or more, of articles in this publication, please contact the Commercial Reprints Department, Elsevier Inc., 360 Park Avenue South, New York, New York 10010-1710. Tel.: (+1) 212-633-3813; Fax: (+1) 212-462-1935 E-mail: reprints@elsevier.com.

The ideas and opinions expressed in *Ultrasound Clinics* do not necessarily reflect those of the Publisher. The Publisher does not assume any responsibility for any injury and/or damage to persons or property arising out of or related to any use of the material contained in this periodical. The reader is advised to check the appropriate medical literature and the product information currently provided by the manufacturer of each drug to be administered to verify the dosage, the method and duration of administration, or contraindications. It is the responsibility of the treating physician or other health care professional, relying on independent experience and knowledge of the patient, to determine drug dosages and the best treatment for the patient. Mention of any product in this issue should not be construed as endorsement by the contributors, editors, or the Publisher of the product or manufacturers' claims.

Ultrasound Clinics (ISSN 1556-858X) is published quarterly by W.B. Saunders, 360 Park Avenue South, New York, NY 10010-1710. Months of publication are January, April, July, and October. Business and editorial offices: 1600 John F. Kennedy Boulevard, Suite 1800, Philadelphia, Pennsylvania 19103-2899. Accounting and circulation offices: 6277 Sea Harbor Drive, Orlando, FL 32887-4800. Periodicals postage paid at New York NY, and additional mailing offices. Subscription prices are USD 175 per year for US individuals, USD 245 per year for US institutions, USD 87 per year for US students and residents, USD 199 per year for Canadian individuals, USD 233 per year for Canadian institutions, USD 199 per year for international individuals, USD 268 per year for international institutions, and USD 99 per year for Canadian and foreign students/residents. To receive student/resident rate, orders must be accompanied by name of affiliated institution, date of term, and the signature of program/residency coordinator on institution letterhead. Orders will be billed at individual rate until proof of status is received. Foreign air speed delivery is included in all Clinics subscription prices. All prices are subject to change without notice. **POSTMASTER:** Send address changes to *Ultrasound Clinics,* Elsevier Periodicals Customer Service, 6277 Sea Harbor Drive, Orlando, FL 32887-4800. **Customer Service: 1-800-654-2452 (US). From outside of the US, call (+1) 407-345-4000.**

Printed in the United States of America.

OBSTETRIC ULTRASOUND/GYNECOLOGIC ULTRASOUND

GUEST EDITORS

DEBORAH LEVINE, MD
Associate Radiologist-in-Chief of Academic Affairs, Co-Chief of Ultrasound, and Director of Ob/Gyn Ultrasound, Department of Radiology, Beth Israel Deaconess Medical Center; and Associate Professor of Radiology, Harvard Medical Center, Boston, Massachusetts

SHEILA SHETH, MD
Associate Professor, Radiology and Pathology, Department of Radiology, School of Medicine, Johns Hopkins University, Baltimore, Maryland

CONTRIBUTORS

TERESITA L. ANGTUACO, MD
Professor of Radiology and Professor of Obstetrics and Gynecology, University of Arkansas for Medical Sciences, Little Rock, Arkansas

OKSANA H. BALTAROWICH, MD
Department of Radiology, Thomas Jefferson University, Philadelphia, Pennsylvania

NIDHI GUPTA, MD
Radiologist-in-Training, Department of Radiology, University of Arkansas for Medical Sciences, Little Rock, Arkansas

MINDY M. HORROW, MD, FACR, FAIUM
Director of Body Imaging, Department of Radiology, Albert Einstein Medical Center; and Associate Professor of Radiology, Jefferson Medical College, Thomas Jefferson University, Philadelphia, Pennsylvania

JOAO FERNANDO KAZAN-TANNUS, MD, PhD
Department of Radiology, Beth Israel Deaconess Medical Center, Boston, Massachusetts

WESLEY LEE, MD, FACOG, FAIUM
Division of Fetal Imaging, William Beaumont Hospital, Royal Oak; Clinical Associate Professor, Department of Obstetrics and Gynecology, Wayne State University, Detroit, Michigan

DEBORAH LEVINE, MD
Associate Radiologist-in-Chief of Academic Affairs, Co-Chief of Ultrasound, and Director of Ob/Gyn Ultrasound, Department of Radiology, Beth Israel Deaconess Medical Center; and Associate Professor of Radiology, Harvard Medical Center, Boston, Massachusetts

ANNA S. LEV-TOAFF, MD
Department of Radiology, Thomas Jefferson University, Philadelphia, Pennsylvania

KATARZYNA MACURA, MD
Assistant Professor, Radiology Diagnostic Imaging, Department of Radiology, School of Medicine, Johns Hopkins University, Baltimore, Maryland

TEJAS S. MEHTA, MD, MPH
Assistant Professor of Radiology, Department of Radiology, Beth Israel Deaconess Medical Center, Boston, Massachusetts

ANA MONTEAGUDO, MD
Professor, Department of Obstetrics & Gynecology, NYU School of Medicine, New York, New York

SHABBIR NAQVI, MD
Department of Radiology, Albert Einstein Medical Center, Philadelphia, Pennsylvania

SHUCHI K. RODGERS, MD
Department of Radiology, Albert Einstein
Medical Center, Philadelphia,
Pennsylvania

LESLIE M. SCOUTT, MD
Department of Diagnostic Radiology, Yale
University School of Medicine, New Haven,
Connecticut

SHEILA SHETH, MD
Associate Professor, Radiology and Pathology,
Department of Radiology, School of Medicine,
Johns Hopkins University, Baltimore, Maryland

ILAN E. TIMOR-TRITSCH, MD
Professor, Department of Obstetrics &
Gynecology, NYU School of Medicine,
New York, New York

OBSTETRIC ULTRASOUND/GYNECOLOGIC ULTRASOUND

Volume 2 • Number 2 • April 2007

Contents

Embryosonology in the First Trimester of Pregnancy 175

Nidhi Gupta and Teresita L. Angtuaco

In the early days of ultrasound, documentation of developmental milestones in the first trimester was limited by the transabdominal approach through a distended urinary bladder. Depiction of the rapid growth and development of the embryo only became possible with the advent of transvaginal sonography in the early 1980s. With better resolution came a clearer correlation between normal embryologic events and ultrasound image displays. Sonographers and sonologists need a clear understanding of the normal sequence of events to distinguish them from abnormal findings. Avoiding pitfalls in diagnosis is necessary to guide management decisions in a patient who presents with first trimester complications.

Ultrasound and MR Imaging of Fetal Neural Tube Defects 187

Tejas S. Mehta and Deborah Levine

Neural tube defects are among the most common congenital anomalies in the United States, the three major types being anencephaly, cephalocele, and spina bifida. By far, most spina bifida cases are myelomeningoceles. Ultrasound plays an important role in the detection and evaluation of these defects. Anencephaly has a characteristic appearance of lack of ossified skull above the orbits, and can be diagnosed in the late first trimester. The spinal defect and brain findings associated with myelomeningocele are well detected by ultrasound, typically in the second trimester. The underlying brain findings in cases of encephalocele are particularly important, and MR imaging is often helpful in these cases. Careful anatomic survey and karyotype analysis are helpful in counseling patients who have a prenatal diagnosis of these defects.

Quantitative Approaches for Volume Sonography During Pregnancy 203

Wesley Lee

As three-dimensional ultrasound imaging technology becomes more widely available, health care providers should understand how software tools can be used to evaluate suspected fetal anomalies. This article summarizes some of the quantitative applications offered by three-dimensional ultrasonography. Volume sonography provides much more than surface and volume-rendered reconstructions of fetal anatomy. Quantitative analysis is now possible by allowing the standardization of distance, angle, area, and volume measurements. Optimal uses of these analytic approaches are emerging as software tools become more sophisticated and as we begin to apply these new capabilities to various clinical problems. Health care providers should be aware of these emerging capabilities and their potential applications.

Ultrasound examination of the fetal central nervous system (CNS) distinguishes itself from the sonographic evaluation of all other organs or organ systems because during the course of pregnancy, the CNS (mainly the fetal brain) undergoes significant changes, in size and in the shape of its different anatomic regions, which follow a well-defined timeline and can be recognized sonographically. The developmental milestones of the CNS from the time of its first sonographic detection to term can, and should, be taken into consideration when a fetal neurosonogram is performed. This article describes a systematic approach to the evaluation of the fetal brain by discussing the differential diagnosis of two important sonographic findings, namely ventriculomegaly and an enlarged posterior fossa, and by touching on other important brain abnormalities.

Fetal tumors have appearances in utero that differ from those seen in neonates and children. Knowledge of these differences is important when assessing a potential fetal neoplasm. Tumors are typically found during routine obstetric ultrasound or in a patient large for dates, either because of the size of the tumor or associated polyhydramnios. After diagnosis, ultrasound is used to follow fetal growth, tumor growth, and any associated abnormalities. Doppler examination is important for differential diagnosis of masses and prediction of outcome. Magnetic resonance imaging frequently adds additional information regarding tissue characterization and organ involvement. The purpose of this review is to describe and illustrate the appearance of fetal tumors with suggestions for differential diagnosis when a fetal mass is visualized.

Pelvic sonography remains the imaging modality of choice for initial evaluation of myometrial pathology. The advent of vaginal sonography and color Doppler sonography have allowed for major refinements in detection and accurate diagnoses of common disorders affecting the uterus, particularly myomas and adenomyosis. Pelvic MR imaging plays an important role in gynecologic imaging because it depicts details of myometrium and junctional zone, is more reproducible, and is less operator-dependent compared with sonography. Because of its higher cost and lesser availability, MR imaging is usually reserved for pretreatment planning and for problem solving in patients for whom the ultrasound is inconclusive, not feasible, or technically suboptimal.

Ultrasound of Pelvic Inflammatory Disease 297

Mindy M. Horrow, Shuchi K. Rodgers, and Shabbir Naqvi

Pelvic sonography is performed commonly in patients who have a clinical diagnosis of pelvic inflammatory disease. Although the study may be normal or sometimes nonspecific, there are various findings that are characteristic of this process. Understanding of the sonographic features of pelvic inflammation, salpingitis, pyosalpinx, tubo–ovarian complex and tubo–ovarian abscess will allow the interpreter to make more specific, clinically useful diagnoses. Sonography also can help to distinguish acute from chronic abnormalities in the fallopian tubes. Correlation of sonography with pelvic CT is important, as CT is ordered with increasing frequency in patients who have unexplained lower abdominal pain

Imaging of Adnexal Torsion 311

Leslie M. Scoutt, Oksana H. Baltarowich, and Anna S. Lev-Toaff

While sudden onset of severe pelvic pain in an afebrile woman of reproductive age is considered the classic presentation of a patient with adnexal torsion, this constellation of findings occurs in the minority of patients with adnexal torsion. In fact, many patients with adnexal torsion present with mild or intermittent symptoms and adnexal torsion likely occurs more frequently than originally thought in post menopausal women. Thus, the clinical presentation is often non-specific and may mimic other gynecologic pathology and even renal or gastrointestinal causes of lower quadrant pain. Duplex Doppler ultrasound (US) is typically the initial imaging study performed in female patients with suspected gynecological pathology. Findings of an enlarged amorphous, heterogenous ovary with an underlying mass or peripheral small follicles in an abnormal midline location are suggestive of ovarian torsion on ultrasound examination. Color Doppler interrogation may demonstrate the twisted blood vessels in the adnexal pedicle. Absence of Doppler detected blood flow suggest torsion and/or infarction but the documentation of blood flow should not exclude the diagnosis of torsion in a painful ovary with suspicious morphologic features. Since computed tomography (CT) may be the first imaging study obtained in patients suspected of harboring gastrointestinal or renal pathology, the radiologist should be familiar with the CT findings or ovarian torsion such as the presence of an enlarged, non-enhancing midline ovary/mass with an adjacent thickened or beak shaped tube or hematoma. Magnetic resonance imaging (MRI) has a role in the work-up of pelvic pain when CT or US findings are non-specific. Findings of adnexal torsion on MR are similar to findings observed on CT. However, the presence of high signal intensity stromal edema and numerous peripheral foillicles as well as lack of stromal enhancement are more easily detected on MRI.

GOAL STATEMENT

The goal of the *Ultrasound Clinics* is to keep practicing radiologists and radiology residents up to date with current clinical practice in ultrasound by providing timely articles reviewing the state of the art in patient care.

ACCREDITATION

The *Ultrasound Clinics* is planned and implemented in accordance with the Essential Areas and Policies of the Accreditation Council for Continuing Medical Education (ACCME) through the joint sponsorship of the University of Virginia School of Medicine and Elsevier. The University of Virginia School of Medicine is accredited by the ACCME to provide continuing medical education for physicians.

The University of Virginia School of Medicine designates this educational activity for a maximum of 15 *AMA PRA Category 1 Credits*™. Physicians should only claim credit commensurate with the extent of their participation in the activity.

The American Medical Association has determined that physicians not licensed in the US who participate in this CME activity are eligible for 15 *AMA PRA Category 1 Credits*™.

Credit can be earned by reading the text material, taking the CME examination online at http://www.theclinics.com/home/cme, and completing the evaluation. After taking the test, you will be required to review any and all incorrect answers. Following completion of the test and evaluation, your credit will be awarded and you may print your certificate.

FACULTY DISCLOSURE/CONFLICT OF INTEREST

The University of Virginia School of Medicine, as an ACCME accredited provider, endorses and strives to comply with the Accreditation Council for Continuing Medical Education (ACCME) Standards of Commercial Support, Commonwealth of Virginia statutes, University of Virginia policies and procedures, and associated federal and private regulations and guidelines on the need for disclosure and monitoring of proprietary and financial interests that may affect the scientific integrity and balance of content delivered in continuing medical education activities under our auspices.

The University of Virginia School of Medicine requires that all CME activities accredited through this institution be developed independently and be scientifically rigorous, balanced and objective in the presentation/discussion of its content, theories and practices.

All authors/editors participating in an accredited CME activity are expected to disclose to the readers relevant financial relationships with commercial entities occurring within the past 12 months (such as grants or research support, employee, consultant, stock holder, member of speakers bureau, etc.). The University of Virginia School of Medicine will employ appropriate mechanisms to resolve potential conflicts of interest to maintain the standards of fair and balanced education to the reader. Questions about specific strategies can be directed to the Office of Continuing Medical Education, University of Virginia School of Medicine, Charlottesville, Virginia.

The authors/editors listed below have identified no professional or financial affiliations for themselves or their spouse/partner:

Teresita L. Angtuaco, MD; Oksana H. Baltarowich, MD; Barton Dudlick (Acquisitions Editor); Nidhi Gupta, MD; Mindy M. Horrow, MD, FACR, FAIUM; Joao Fernando Kazan-Tannus, MD, PhD; Deborah Levine, MD (Guest Editor); Anna S. Lev-Toaff, MD; Katarzyna Macura, MD; Tejas S. Mehta, MD, MPH; Ana Monteagudo, MD; Shabbir Naqvi, MD; Shuchi K. Rodgers, MD; Leslie M. Scoutt, MD; and, Sheila Sheth, MD (Guest Editor).

The authors/editors listed below have identified the following professional or financial affiliations for themselves or their spouse/partner:

Wesley Lee, MD, FACOG, FAIUM is a consultant and has received research support from Siemens and Phillips; is a consultant, speaker, and has received research support from GE Healthcare.
Ilan E. Timor-Tritsch, MD is a consultant for GE Healthcare.

Disclosure of Discussion of non-FDA approved uses for pharmaceutical products and/or medical devices:
The University of Virginia School of Medicine, as an ACCME provider, requires that all faculty presenters identify and disclose any "off label" uses for pharmaceutical and medical device products. The University of Virginia School of Medicine recommends that each physician fully review all the available data on new products or procedures prior to instituting them with patients.

TO ENROLL

To enroll in the Ultrasound Clinics Continuing Medical Education program, call customer service at 1-800-654-2452 or visit us online at www.theclinics.com/home/cme. The CME program is available to subscribers for an additional fee of $205.00.

FORTHCOMING ISSUES

RECENT ISSUES

THE CLINICS ARE NOW AVAILABLE ONLINE!

Access your subscription at:
www.theclinics.com

ULTRASOUND
CLINICS

Ultrasound Clin 2 (2007) xi

Preface

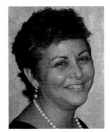

Deborah Levine, MD
Guest Editor

Deborah Levine, MD
Department of Radiology
Beth Israel Deaconess Medical Center
330 Brookline Avenue
Boston, MA 02215, USA

E-mail address:
dlevine@bidmc.harvard.edu

It is with great pleasure that I write this introduction to the second issue on Obstetric Ultrasound for *Ultrasound Clinics*. The editors have assembled articles that will be of interest to obstetricians, gynecologists, sonographers, and radiologists.

In the first section, there is an article on embryosonology by Drs. Gupta and Angtuaco. This article gives a fine review of the imaging appearance of normal early pregnancy with respect to the sequence of embryonologic events that occur during this time. There are two articles that describe assessment of the fetal central nervous system. Drs. Monteagudo and Timor-Tritsch give detailed illustrations of the dedicated scan of the fetal brain. They illustrate the normal and abnormal appearance of the fetal brain throughout gestation, and give detailed descriptions of scanning in 2D and 3D. Dr. Mehta reviews imaging of fetal neural tube defects, including encephaloceles, anencephaly, and spinal neural tube defects, showing correlative

imaging with ultrasound and MR imaging. Dr. Lee's article on quantitative approaches for volume sonography during pregnancy reviews basic approaches for the quantitative analysis, including technical aspects of scanning and assessments of volumes. He illustrates how quantitative analysis can be useful for assessment of fetal abnormalities, such as pulmonary hypoplasia, chromosomal anomalies, and micrognathia. Finally, a review by Dr. Kazan Tannus details the sonographic and magnetic resonance appearance of a wide variety of fetal tumors, and gives a structured differential diagnosis for tumors in various locations in the fetal body.

As evidenced by this overview, this issue has articles that span all three trimesters and combine 2D and 3D ultrasound, as well as fetal magnetic resonance imaging. I hope this issue of *Clinics* will aid prenatal diagnosticians in their pursuit of quality fetal ultrasound.

ultrasound.theclinics.com

doi:10.1016/j.cult.2007.11.001

ULTRASOUND
CLINICS

Ultrasound Clin 2 (2007) 175–185

Embryosonology in the First Trimester of Pregnancy

Nidhi Gupta, MD[a],*, Teresita L. Angtuaco, MD[b]

- Conceptus period (3–5 weeks menstrual age)
- Embryonic period (6–9 weeks)
- Fetal period (10–12 weeks)
- Summary
- References

The first trimester of pregnancy is defined as the 13 weeks following the first day of the last menstrual period (LMP). Although the actual gestational age begins at fertilization, most imaging references to developmental milestones are based on menstrual weeks. As such, all references to embryonic or fetal age in this review are expressed in menstrual weeks.

Since the establishment of ultrasound as the primary diagnostic test in pregnancy, a wide spectrum of sonographic findings seen during the first trimester have been described in the literature. To recognize normal and abnormal early pregnancy development, one must have a thorough knowledge of the embryologic sequence of events that lead to the completion of the first trimester of gestation. Embryologically the first 1 to 2 weeks of the first trimester is called the ovarian period. This is followed by the conceptus period (3–5 weeks menstrual age), the embryonic period (6–10 weeks), and the fetal period (11–12 weeks) [1]. The ovarian period spans the time from menses to ovulation and therefore is not treated separately in this review.

Conceptus period (3–5 weeks menstrual age)

Human development begins with fertilization and formation of the zygote. As the zygote passes along the fallopian tube toward the uterus, it undergoes cleavage into several smaller cells termed blastomeres. Approximately 3 days after fertilization a ball of 12 or more blastomeres forms the morula and enters the uterus. A cavity soon forms within the morula converting it into a blastocyst (Fig. 1). The blastocyst is composed of three components: the embryoblast, which gives rise to the embryo and some extraembryonic structures, the blastocystic cavity, and the trophoblast, a thin outer layer of cells that forms extraembryonic structures and the embryonic part of the placenta. By the end of the first week of fertilization (third menstrual week), the blastocyst is superficially implanted in the endometrium [2]. During the fourth menstrual week, the blastocyst completes its implantation into the endometrium, which is now referred to as the decidua. The primary yolk sac forms and gradually disappears as the secondary yolk sac develops at 27 to 28 menstrual days (Fig. 2). It is the secondary rather than the primary yolk sac that is visible with ultrasound. During the fifth menstrual week, the coelomic cavity within the embryo arises and eventually forms the body cavities.

Sonographically the endometrial changes that occur can be characterized during this time. There have been several studies regarding characteristics

[a] Department of Radiology #556, University of Arkansas for Medical Sciences, 4301 West Markham 2, Little Rock, AR 72205, USA
[b] Obstetrics and Gynecology, University of Arkansas for Medical Sciences, 4301 W. Markham 2, Little Rock, AR 72205, USA
* Corresponding author.
E-mail address: nidigupta@yahoo.com (N. Gupta).

1556-858X/07/$ – see front matter © 2007 Elsevier Inc. All rights reserved.
ultrasound.theclinics.com
doi:10.1016/j.cult.2007.07.006

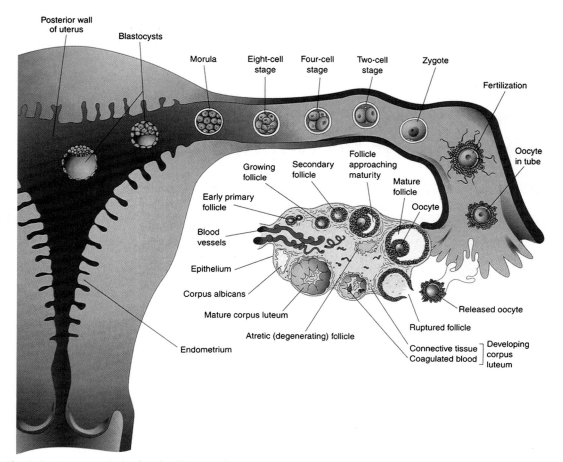

Fig. 1. Conceptus period. After fertilization the zygote undergoes a series of transformation and implants in the decidua as a blastocyst. (*Reproduced from* Moore KL, Persaud TVN. The developing human: clinically oriented embryology. 7th edition. Philadelphia: Saunders; 2003. p. 1–117; with permission.)

that would predict endometrial receptivity and successful implantation in pregnancy. Currently there is reasonable certainty that women who have heterogeneous endometrial linings less than 6 mm rarely conceive [3]. Optimal conditions of implantation have been described in the literature, such as endometrial thickness greater than 7 mm (Fig. 3) and hypoechogenic endometrium with five well-defined layers on high-resolution sonography. Also, Doppler visualization of subendometrial flow is a good prognostic indicator. Pulsatility index (PI) values of 3 or higher usually indicate poor outcome [4].

Before a yolk sac or embryo can be visualized, an intrauterine fluid collection is often seen (Fig. 4). It is important to determine if this intrauterine fluid collection represents an intrauterine pregnancy (IUP), a pseudogestational sac associated with an ectopic pregnancy, or a decidual cyst that, although associated with ectopic pregnancy, can also be seen in IUP. Several signs have been suggested to

distinguish these possibilities. In 1982 Bradley and colleagues [5] described "the double decidual sac sign" (Fig. 5). This was described as two concentric echogenic rings of tissue surrounding the intrauterine sac that protrudes into the uterine cavity. This morphologic appearance differs from the pseudosac of an ectopic pregnancy and virtually excludes its presence. The two concentric rings represent the apposing surfaces of the decidua capsularis that surrounds the developing gestational sac and the decidua parietalis (decidua vera) that lines the uterine wall on the opposite side of the implantation site. After this sign was described it was realized that a yolk sac was typically present by the time the double decidual sac sign can be properly visualized. Because of this time frame, the usefulness of the double decidual sac sign has been questioned.

In 1988 Yeh [6] described the intradecidual sign. This term refers to an echogenic area representing the implanted blastocyst that is embedded in the

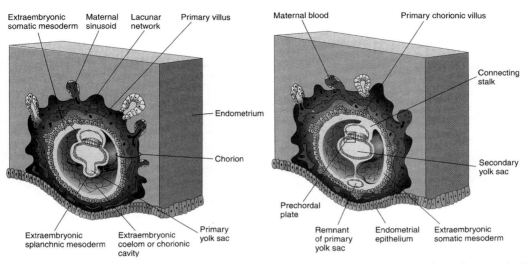

Fig. 2. Primary and secondary yolk sac. At approximately 28 menstrual days, the primary yolk sac decreases in size as the secondary yolk sac is formed. It is the secondary yolk sac that becomes visible on ultrasound. (*Reproduced from* Moore KL, Persaud TVN. The developing human: clinically oriented embryology. 7th edition. Philadelphia: Saunders; 2003. p. 1–117; with permission.)

thickened decidua and thus is eccentrically located on one side of the uterine cavity. As the gestational sac grows, the echogenic area becomes a well-defined cystic cavity. This eccentric location is caused by the developing gestational sac burrowing into the decidua as it establishes its own blood supply. The true uterine cavity therefore is seen separately as a well-defined endometrial stripe that is often indented by the developing gestational sac (Fig. 6). This finding is crucial in distinguishing it from the pseudogestational sac of an ectopic pregnancy, which appears as fluid surrounded by the echogenic endometrial lining. Yeh and colleagues reported

that the intradecidual sign was shown to reveal implantation as early as 25 days after fertilization, earlier than the effective window for the double decidual sac sign, and was more specific and sensitive in detecting early IUP. Another recent study by Chiang and colleagues [7] concluded that the intradecidual sign reliably excludes the presence of an ectopic pregnancy. The accuracy for diagnosis of an IUP increases when this sign is associated with serum beta human chorionic gonadotropin (HCG) levels equal to or greater than 2000 mIU/mL or

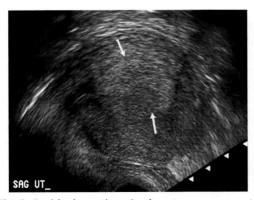

Fig. 3. Decidual reaction. As the uterus prepares to receive the blastocyst, the endometrium (*arrows*) becomes thickened and hypoechoic. An endometrial thickness of at least 7 mm provides an optimum condition for implantation.

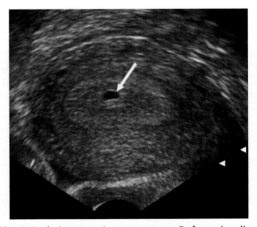

Fig. 4. Early intrauterine pregnancy. Before visualization of the yolk sac or embryo, the earliest sign of pregnancy is an intrauterine fluid collection (*arrow*) that needs to be distinguished from the decidual cast of an ectopic pregnancy.

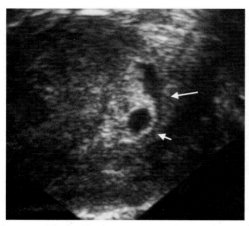

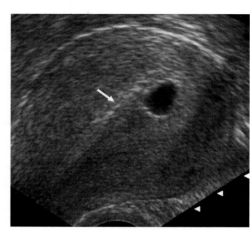

Fig. 5. Double decidual sac sign. Two layers of decidua are separated by fluid in the uterine cavity. The decidua capsularis (*short arrow*) surrounds the developing gestational sac, and the decidua parietalis (*long arrow*) is seen on the opposite wall of the uterus.

Fig. 6. Intradecidual sign. The gestational sac is implanted on one side of the decidua, giving an eccentric location relative to the uterine cavity (*arrow*). The linear endometrial cavity should be defined surrounding the gestational sac to establish this sign.

a mean sac diameter equal to or greater than 3 mm. It is of utmost importance to visualize this sign on multiple views with an unchanging appearance.

With endovaginal sonography, the gestational sac may be seen within the decidua at approximately 4.5 weeks menstrual age. The gestational sac is an anechoic space surrounded by a hyperechoic rim of trophoblastic tissue. Before other structures are visualized in the gestational sac, it is the only means of estimating gestational age and can therefore be measured. The mean sac diameter (MSD) is obtained by averaging three orthogonal measurements. The anteroposterior and cephalocaudad measurements are obtained on a sagittal (longitudinal) view and the transverse diameter is obtained on an axial view (Fig. 7). This technique avoids

the erroneous enlargement of the anteroposterior view when it is obtained on the axial view. In this case, the transducer may be lined up in an oblique plane causing the false measurement. The MSD grows in a linear fashion. The range of precision for a first-trimester parameter is plus or minus 1 week (2 standard deviations [SD]) [8].

The yolk sac is the first structure to be seen within the gestational sac (Figs. 8 and 9) and confirms the presence of a gestational sac rather than a decidual cast or pseudogestational sac [9]. Using transabdominal sonography, the yolk sac is often seen at MSD of approximately 10 to 15 mm and should always be visualized by MSD of 20 mm. By transvaginal ultrasound, yolk sac is usually visualized by MSD of 8 to 10 mm [10]. The upper limit of normal for

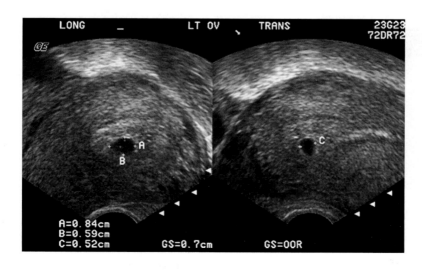

Fig. 7. Gestational sac measurement. This earliest measurement for determining the gestational age is obtained by taking the mean of three diameters. The cephalocaudad and anteroposterior diameters are taken on the sagittal view and the transverse measurement on the coronal view.

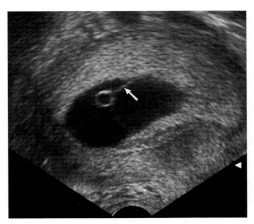

Fig. 8. Yolk sac. The first confirmatory sign of an intra-uterine gestation is the visualization of the secondary yolk sac, which is often seen attached to a stalk (*arrow*).

yolk sac diameter between 5 and 10 weeks menstrual age is 5.6 mm. In addition, the number of yolk sacs can be helpful in determining amnionicity of the pregnancy. The amnion and yolk sac differentiate at approximately the same time, but the yolk sac is more readily visible on sonography than the thin amniotic membrane. Even if the amniotic membrane is not well visualized on sonography, the presence of two yolk sacs therefore implies two amniotic sacs (Fig. 10) [11]. One of the earliest pieces of evidence of an embryo has also been described as the double-bleb sign. This sign has the appearance of two small bubbles (amniotic and yolk sacs) attached to the wall of the gestational sac (Fig. 11). The embryonic disc is located between the two bubbles. This is a transient phenomenon and is the least observed of all the early signs of a normal pregnancy [12]. The observation of all

these signs of pregnancy is predicated on the endovaginal visualization of a yolk sac by MSD of 10 mm and an embryo at MSD of 15 mm. It is therefore suggested that an MSD greater than 16 mm without an embryo indicates a nonviable pregnancy (Fig. 12) [6]. This is most often caused by an anembryonic pregnancy in which the gestational sac development was progressing normally but the embryo never materializes, or an embryo developed and then was reabsorbed Sonographically this may be indistinguishable from an incomplete abortion, but clinically there is no sign of external bleeding in anembryonic gestation. In the old literature this finding was termed blighted ovum because of the erroneous belief that pregnancy failure was only caused by deficiencies associated with the ovum. The change in terminology reflects the recognition that this event is multifactorial in etiology. Although the MSD of 16 mm has been cited as the measurement at which an abnormal pregnancy is suspected, in actual practice it is best to give the pregnancy the benefit of the doubt and allow a few millimeters technical allowance rather than have rigid sets of rules. When the MSD is in the borderline range, it is wise to correlate with serial HCG levels (which, if declining, indicate a nonviable pregnancy) or to do a follow-up examination to determine the presence or absence of growth of the sac, the development of a yolk sac/embryo, and the visualization of a heart beat.

Embryonic period (6–9 weeks)

Major changes occur in body form beginning at 6 menstrual weeks. Essentially all internal and external structures present in the adult form during the embryonic period. By the end of the sixth week blood flow is unidirectional, and by the end of

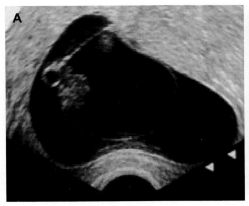

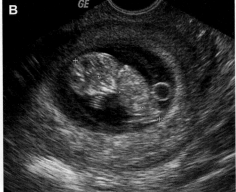

Fig. 9. Yolk sac on endovaginal images. The appearance of the amniotic membrane defines the extra-amniotic location of the yolk sac.

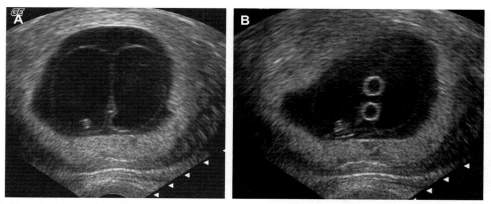

Fig. 10. Diamniotic gestation. The presence of two amniotic cavities is implied by the visualization of two yolk sacs even when the twin embryos are not seen.

the eighth week the heart attains its definite form. The peripheral vascular system develops a little later and is completed by the end of the tenth week (Fig. 13). The primitive gut forms during the sixth week. The midgut herniates into the umbilical cord beginning from the eighth week until the end of the twelfth week (Fig. 14). This is caused by the inability of the abdomen to accommodate the rapidly growing small bowel. The temporary herniation slowly resolves as the gut returns to the expanding abdominal cavity. This normal phenomenon is not seen beyond the first trimester. The rectum separates from the urogenital sinus by the end of week 8, and the anal membrane perforates by the end of week 10. The metanephros, or primitive kidneys, ascend from the pelvis starting at approximately week 8, but do not reach their adult position until week 11. Limbs are formed with

separate fingers and toes. Nearly all congenital malformations except for abnormalities of the genitalia originate before or during the embryonic period. External genitalia are still in a sexless state at the end of week 10 and do not reach mature fetal form until the end of week 14 [13].

Sonographically, cardiac activity can be identified as early as 34 days and at a crown–rump length (CRL) of 1 to 2 mm [14]. On endovaginal sonography, absent cardiac activity in an embryo having a CRL of greater than 5 mm indicates embryonic demise (Fig. 15) [9]. In addition, the number and the clarity of structures increase from 7 to 8 weeks of gestation. At 8 weeks secondary brain vesicles, spine, liver, upper and lower limb buds, and sacral tail can be visualized in all fetuses. The four-chamber view can be identified at 8 weeks, as can fingers or toes. The stomach can be first noted at 9 weeks

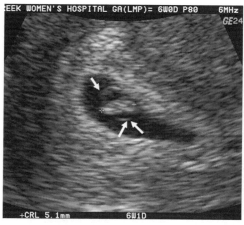

Fig. 11. Double bleb sign. The yolk sac (*arrow*) and the enlarging amniotic cavity (*double arrows*) form the two blebs that surround the embryo in this 6-week gestation.

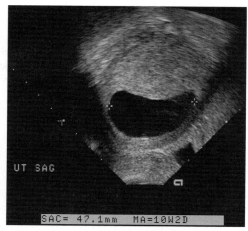

Fig. 12. Anembryonic gestation. A gestational sac measuring greater than 20 mm (MSD) without an embryo should be considered abnormal.

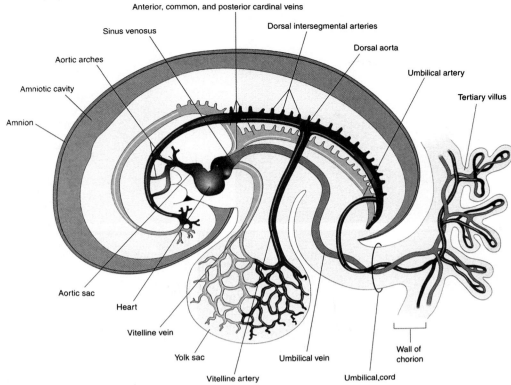

Fig. 13. Cardiovascular system of the embryo. At approximately 35 menstrual days, the vascular system of the embryo is established between the chorionic villi and the yolk sac. Oxygenated blood from the villi is brought back to the embryo by the umbilical vein. (*Reproduced from* Moore KL, Persaud TVN. The developing human: clinically oriented embryology. 7th edition. Philadelphia: Saunders; 2003. p. 1–117; with permission.)

[15]. Physiologic midgut herniation can be visualized at 8 to 12 weeks as a local bulge at the cord insertion. At 12 completed weeks, the gut retracts into the abdominal cavity [16,17]. Early detection of major fetal anomalies such as anencephaly and anterior abdominal wall defects is therefore possible at this early stage.

The open rhombencephalon is an important finding that was first reported by Cyr and colleagues [13]. This is seen at 8 to 10 menstrual weeks and manifests as a small cystic structure (3–4 mm) in the posterior aspect of the cranium, which eventually develops into the normally proportioned fourth ventricle after the eleventh menstrual week (Fig. 16). Recognition of this as a normal finding is important so as not to make the wrong diagnosis of brain anomalies. When in doubt, a follow-up examination at the end of the first trimester shows the disappearance of the cystic structure that is now covered by the normally formed cerebellum.

Of the various measurements used for estimating fetal gestational age, measurement of CRL is the method of choice during first trimester [2]. A well-performed CRL measurement in the first trimester

of pregnancy is accurate within 5 to 7days [14]. This is still the most reliable of all sonographic parameters for dating purposes. It is therefore important that the CRL be measured accurately (Fig. 17). Usually the measurement is obtained using endovaginal sonography and the image magnified for proper placement of the calipers. Later in the first trimester, the fetus should be slightly flexed and not extended during measurement. The maximum length should be measured and compared with existing tables for proper dating (Fig. 18).

Fetal period (10–12 weeks)

At the beginning of the tenth week the head constitutes a large proportion of the CRL of the fetus. From 10 weeks, growth in body length accelerates rapidly, and by the end of 12 weeks the CRL has more than doubled. Although the growth of the head slows considerably by the twelfth week, it is still disproportionately large compared with the rest of the body. In addition, at the end of 12 weeks, primary ossification centers appear in the skeleton,

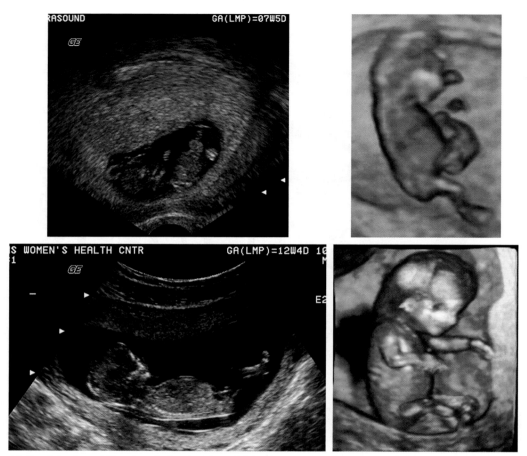

Fig. 14. Physiologic umbilical herniation in 2-D and 3-D. The transient herniation of the small bowel at the base of the umbilical cord insertion is seen in the 7-week embryo (*arrow*) and resolved in the 12-week fetus.

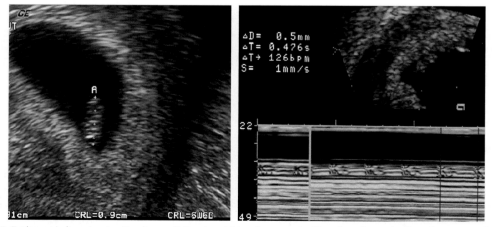

Fig. 15. Embryonic heart rate. Cardiac activity should be documented in all embryos longer than 5 mm by CRL. A normal rate of at least 110/min should be recorded.

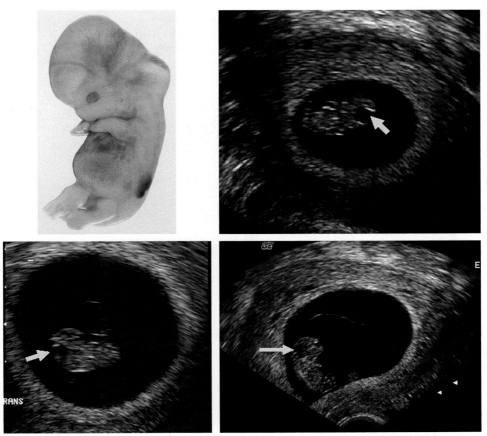

Fig. 16. Open rhombencephalon. The fourth ventricle in the posterior fossa manifests as a cystic mass (*arrow*) that bulges out of the occipital pole of the embryo. This is usually seen at 8 to 10 weeks and resolves by 12 weeks as the cerebellum forms a roof over it. Varying sizes and degrees of prominence of the cystic mass are demonstrated.

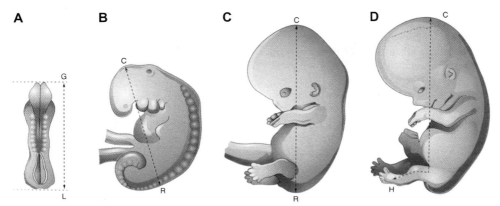

Fig. 17. Embryonic measurements. (*A,B*) Measurements of the greatest length of the embryo before discernment of the head and rump. (*C*) CRL. (*D*) Crown–heel length. (*Reproduced from* Moore KL, Persaud TVN. The developing human: clinically oriented embryology. 7th edition. Philadelphia: Saunders; 2003. p. 1–117; with permission.)

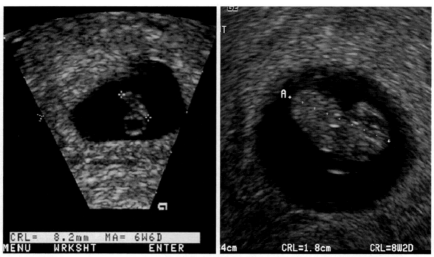

Fig. 18. Embryonic measurements. The greatest length measurement at 6 weeks is usually referred to as crown–rump length even though the crown and the rump may not be as clearly defined as at 8 weeks.

especially in the skull and the long bones. By the end of the twelfth week the upper extremities have reached their final relative length, whereas the lower extremities are still not well developed and are slightly shorter than their final relative length. It is at this stage of pregnancy that the distinctive features of the fetus can be readily appreciated by the parents and bonding can begin. Active fetal movements that can be seen on the ultrasound screen but not yet felt become a source of fascination for the mother who wonders at such activity. It is from this point on that the fetus starts to grow and mature until term.

Summary

The first trimester begins with two cells at fertilization and ends with a developed fetus at 13 weeks. Ultrasound's ability to witness each phase of this evolution can create diagnostic dilemmas among those not familiar with the sequence of events that this rapid transformation entails. Knowledge of embryology is essential in differentiating normal from abnormal findings. Different signs have been described in the first 5 menstrual weeks to ascertain whether the intrauterine changes indicate the presence of an IUP. Once the presence of pregnancy is ascertained, follow-up of the developing gestational sac, embryo, and fetus provide key findings to help determine if there is a normal progression of pregnancy. Any aberration in the developmental process during organogenesis allows the identification of anomalies as early as 9 weeks [2].

References

[1] Sohaey R, Woodward P. The spectrum of first-trimester ultrasound findings. Curr Probl Diagn Radiol 1996;25(2):54–75.

[2] Moore KL, Persaud TVN. The developing human: clinically oriented embryology. 7th edition. Philadelphia: Saunders; 2003. p. 1–117.

[3] Pierson RA. Imaging the endometrium: are there predictors of uterine receptivity? J Obstet Gynaecol Can 2003;25(5):360–8.

[4] Damon VB, Bessai K, Gregor J. [Using ultrasound imaging in implantation]. Zentralbl Gynakol 2001;123(6):340–3 [in German].

[5] Bradley WG, Fiske CE, Filly RA. The double sac sign of early intrauterine pregnancy: use in exclusion of ectopic pregnancy. Radiology 1982; 143(1):223–6.

[6] Yeh HC. Sonographic signs of early pregnancy. Crit Rev Diagn Imaging 1988;28(3): 181–211.

[7] Chiang G, Levine D, Swire M, et al. The intradecidual sign: is it reliable for diagnosis of early intrauterine pregnancy? AJR Am J Roentgenol 2004;183(3):725–31.

[8] Middleton WD, Alfred BK, Barbara SH. The first trimester and ectopic pregnancy. In: The requisites: ultrasound. 3rd edition. St. Louis (MO): Mosby; 2004. p. 342–73.

[9] Levi CS, Lyons EA, Lindsay DJ. Ultrasound in the first trimester of pregnancy. Radiol Clin North Am 1990;28(1):19–38.

[10] Nyberg DA, Mack LA, Laing FC, et al. Distinguishing normal from abnormal gestational sac growth in early pregnancy. J Ultrasound Med 1987;6(1):23–7.

[11] Lindsay DJ, Lovett IS, Lyons EA, et al. Yolk sac diameter and shape at endovaginal US: predictors

of pregnancy outcome in the first trimester. Radiology 1992;183(1):115–8.

[12] Yeh HC, Rabinowitz JG. Amniotic sac development: ultrasound features of early pregnancy—the double bleb sign. Radiology 1988;166(1 Pt 1): 97–103.

[13] Cyr DR, Mack LA, Nyberg DA, et al. Fetal rhombencephalon: normal US findings. Radiology 1988;166(3):691–2.

[14] Lyons EA, Levi CS. The first trimester. In: Rumack CM, Wilson SR, Charboneau JW, et al, editors. Diagnostic ultrasound. 3rd edition. St. Louis (MO): Elseivier Mosby; 2005. p. 1069–126.

[15] Britten S, Soenksen DM, Bustillo M, et al. Very early (24-56 days from last menstrual period) embryonic heart rate in normal pregnancies. Hum Reprod 1994;9(12):2424–6.

[16] Fujiwaki R, Hata T, Hata K, et al. Intrauterine ultrasonographic assessments of embryonic development. Am J Obstet Gynecol 1995;173(6): 1770–4.

[17] Blaas HG, Eik-Nes SH, Kiserud T, et al. Early development of the abdominal wall, stomach and heart from 7 to 12 weeks of gestation: a longitudinal ultrasound study. Ultrasound Obstet Gynecol 1995;6(4):240–9.

ELSEVIER
SAUNDERS

ULTRASOUND CLINICS

Ultrasound Clin 2 (2007) 187–201

Ultrasound and MR Imaging of Fetal Neural Tube Defects

Tejas S. Mehta, MD, MPH*, Deborah Levine, MD

Neural tube defects (NTDs) are among the most common congenital anomalies in the United States, occurring at a rate of 1 to 2 cases per 1000 births [1,2]. The three major types of NTDs are anencephaly, cephalocele, and spina bifida. The incidence of NTDs varies with ethnicity, geographic location, and socioeconomic status [3–5]. The causes of NTDs are also varied, with most (up to 88%) being isolated and multifactorial [6–8]. Chromosomal abnormalities, maternal diseases such as type 1 diabetes mellitus, fetal exposure to teratogens such as anticonvulsants, and amniotic band syndrome are other less common causes of NTDs [2,6,8–12]. Because of these associations, when an NTD is seen sonographically, a careful fetal anatomic survey is performed to evaluate for associated anomalies. Because associated chromosomal anomalies have been reported in up to 16% with even isolated NTDs, amniocentesis is typically recommended [13,14]. Women with a history of prior pregnancy with NTD are advised to take higher doses of folic acid supplements, compared with the general population. Folic acid during pregnancy has been shown to be

protective in these patients, decreasing the risk of recurrence.

Spinal neural tube defects

Spina bifida is categorized by its contents; more than 90% of the cases are myelomeningocele (containing neural elements), with the remainder being meningocele (containing no neural elements). Spina bifida can also be characterized as an "open" defect (80%) or a "closed" defect (20%). Lesions may occur anywhere along the spine, but are most common in the lumbar and sacral regions.

Many have proposed that, with the advances in technology, in experienced hands, and with the knowledge of the cranial findings associated with NTDs, ultrasound is a better screening test for NTDs than maternal serum alpha-fetoprotein (MSAFP). Using a threshold of 2.5 multiples of the median for singleton pregnancies, MSAFP detects 80% of fetuses with open spina bifida, with a false-positive rate of 4% [15]. Ultrasound has reported sensitivities ranging from 96% to 100%, with specificity of 100% [16–19].

Department of Radiology, Beth Israel Deaconess Medical Center, 330 Brookline Avenue, Boston, MA 02215, USA
* Corresponding author.
E-mail address: tmehta@bidmc.harvard.edu (T.S. Mehta).

1556-858X/07/$ – see front matter © 2007 Elsevier Inc. All rights reserved.
ultrasound.theclinics.com

doi:10.1016/j.cult.2007.07.005

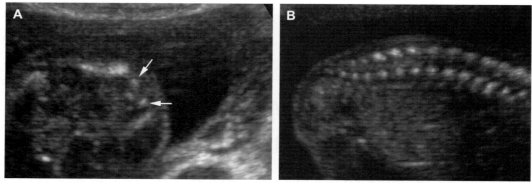

Fig. 1. Normal views of the distal spine in a fetus at 19 weeks. (*A*) The posterior elements angle toward each other on the transverse view (*arrows*). (*B*) The spinal elements converge and have a gentle upward turn on the sagittal view.

Spinal findings

The most common type of spina bifida is a myelomeningocele. The American Institute of Ultrasound in Medicine, the American College of Radiology, and the American College of Obstetrics and Gynecology guidelines for obstetric ultrasound [20] require views of the spine. The spine is evaluated in the sagittal and axial planes in the cervical,

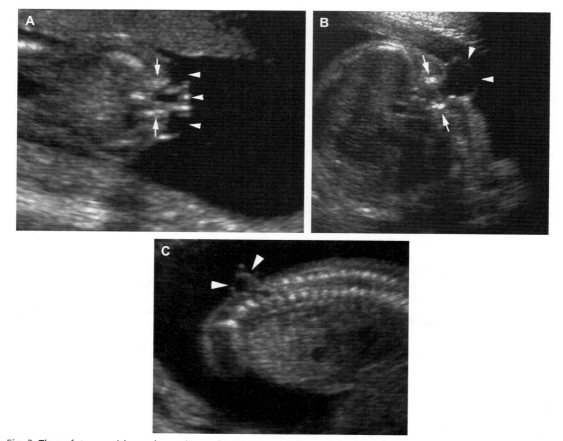

Fig. 2. Three fetuses with myelomeningoceles. Transverse views of the lumbar region in a fetus at 19 weeks (*A*) and of the thoracic region in a fetus at 29 weeks (*B*). Note the nonconvergence of the posterior elements (*arrows*) and the posterior cystic region (*arrowheads*). (*C*) Sagittal view of a fetus at 18 weeks shows spinal defect with a cystic region (*arrowheads*).

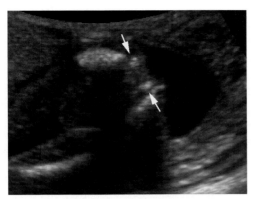

Fig. 3. Transverse view of the distal spine in a fetus at 19 weeks with myelomeningocele shows nonconvergence of the posterior elements (*arrows*). A posterior sac is not seen.

thoracic, lumbar, and sacral regions. Because NTDs are most common in the lumbosacral spine, particular attention is paid to the distal spine. Three ossification centers are located in the fetal vertebrae, one in the body and one at the base of each transverse process. On a transverse view, the posterior elements are seen as "parallel" bands of echoes that flare in the upper cervical spine and converge in the sacrum [21]. In the normal fetus, on the transverse view of the distal spine, the posterior elements should be parallel or angle toward one another. On the sagittal view, the spinal elements should be parallel, should converge, and should have a gentle upward turn (Fig. 1). The distal spine may not ossify before 22 weeks gestation [22,23]. In the second trimester, the lowest ossification center typically visualized is at the level of the third sacral vertebral body (S3), and in the third trimester at the level of the fourth sacral vertebral body (S4), which limits

the sonographic evaluation of the distal sacral spine in the early second trimester, because the lower vertebral bodies may be incompletely ossified.

With a myelomeningocele, there is loss of the posterior overlying soft tissue with the presence of a cystic lesion (Fig. 2). At times, only the nonconvergence or splaying of the posterior elements will be visible (Fig. 3). In the transverse plane, the lateral processes are splayed, with the ossification centers being further apart than those above or below the defect. One may see a cleft in the soft tissues and a cyst protruding posteriorly. Care should be taken not to have too much craniocaudal angulation in the transverse projection, because this angulation can give the appearance of splaying or "pseudodysraphism" in an otherwise normal fetus [24]. It is possible to make a normal distal spine appear to have nonconvergence of the posterior elements. It is therefore important to scan above and below the area in question, to ensure that the nonconvergence is a real finding. The coronal plane shows lateral displacement and widening of the otherwise parallel echogenic lateral processes (Fig. 4). The level of the NTD should be estimated because it is associated with prognosis. The last rib is used as a marker for T12. Vertebral bodies are counted above or below this, as appropriate. The last ossified vertebral body (which depends on gestational age, as discussed previously) can also be used, as can the level of the sacrum at S1.

Fetal scoliosis is also associated with myelomeningoceles (Fig. 5). Thus, any fetus with an apparent isolated scoliosis should be carefully assessed for other signs of NTD. In one study of 20 fetuses with scoliosis, 60% were associated with NTDs [25]. The presence of scoliosis can make determining the level of the defect more difficult.

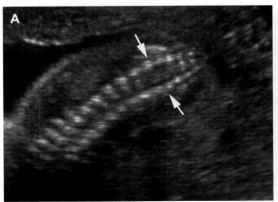
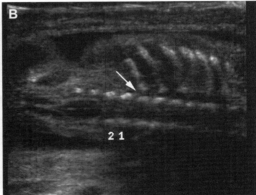

Fig. 4. Coronal views of the spine in two fetuses with myelomeningoceles. (*A*) Fetus at 20 weeks gestation shows subtle lateral displacement of the posterior elements in the lumbar spine (*arrows*), which then reconverge toward the distal sacral spine. (*B*) Fetus at 17 weeks gestation. This view is helpful in determining the level of the defect, an important prognostic indicator, by identifying the vertebral body with the last rib (*arrow*) as T12, and counting inferiorly. In this case, the splaying of the posterior elements starts at L1. 1, L1 vertebral body; 2, L2 vertebral body.

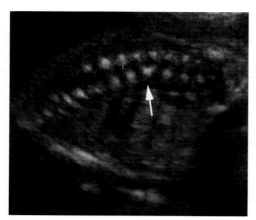

Fig. 5. Sagittal oblique view of a fetus at 15 weeks with NTD (not shown in this image) and scoliosis. Note the sharp angulation of the spine (*arrow*).

Cranial findings of spinal neural tube defects

The three main sonographic cranial findings associated with NTDs are

1. Arnold-Chiari (Chiari II) malformation with banana-shaped cerebellum and effacement of the cisterna magna
2. Lemon configuration to the skull
3. Ventriculomegaly

Less common cranial findings include a small biparietal diameter (BPD) and a small transcerebellar diameter (TCD) [16,26–35]. In a study of 234 fetuses with spina bifida examined before 24 weeks, all but 2 (99%) had at least one of the above cranial findings [15]. Obstetric imaging guidelines require views of the head at the level of the BPD, lateral ventricles, and cerebellum, which show abnormalities such as ventriculomegaly, lemon-shaped skull, and Chiari II malformation [20].

Because most open NTDs are associated with Chiari II malformations, the sonographic diagnosis depends not only on the spinal findings but also on the cranial findings, which is of critical importance in the evaluation of distal NTDs because, as mentioned previously, the spine may not be completely ossified in the early second trimester. Often, it is the posterior fossa findings that indicate that a NTD is present. The hallmark of the Chiari II malformation is dysgenesis of the hindbrain with caudal displacement of the fourth ventricle and brainstem, and tonsillar and vermian herniation through the foramen magnum. Nicolaides and colleagues [26] described the banana sign in association with spina bifida, which is caused by the Chiari II malformation.

Normally, the cerebellum has the configuration of a "3" (Fig. 6). In Chiari II malformation the cerebellum is displaced caudally, which can cause a change in configuration of the cerebellum to

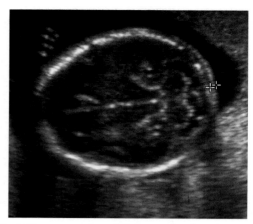

Fig. 6. Transverse view of the posterior fossa in a normal fetus at 18 weeks gestation. The cerebellum has a normal shape of a "3." Calipers mark the nuchal fold thickness. The cisterna magna is normal.

resemble a banana (Fig. 7) and efface the cisterna magna such that it measures less than 2 mm in diameter [26,28,30,36]. It has been reported that this inferior displacement of the brain is caused by a decrease in intraspinal pressure or tethering of the spinal cord [37]. Thus, early in gestation, the cerebellum may look normal [34,37], with eventual appearance of the banana sign, and evolution of an obliterated cisterna magna [16]. This downward displacement is also felt to play a role in the development of ventriculomegaly, by way of the mechanism of obstruction of cerebrospinal fluid [38]. The Chiari II malformation is almost always associated with either a spinal or cranial NTD. In rare instances, an effaced cisterna magna is seen in cases of ventriculomegaly without NTD. A normal-appearing cisterna

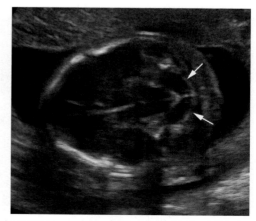

Fig. 7. Transverse view of the posterior fossa in a fetus with NTD at 19 weeks gestation. The cerebellum (*arrows*) is wrapped around the midbrain, resulting in the appearance of a "banana." The cisterna magna is effaced and cannot be measured.

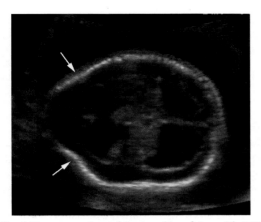

Fig. 8. Transverse view of the head in a fetus with NTD at 19 weeks gestation shows marked concavity of the frontal bones (*arrows*), known as the "lemon" sign. Associated ventriculomegaly is also noted.

magna has a high negative predictive value in the assessment for NTDs [30].

Nicolaides and colleagues [26] were the first to describe the lemon sign in association with fetuses with spina bifida (Fig. 8). This sign is a concave deformity of the frontal bones best seen at the level of the lateral ventricles, although it can also be seen at the level of the thalami and cavum septi pellucidi (at the level of the BPD) [31]. The lemon sign is not specific for spina bifida; it can be seen with encephaloceles [39], and in 1% of the normal population [19,31,40]. Thus, the positive predictive value of the lemon sign for spina bifida depends on the prevalence of spina bifida in the population [40]. The lemon sign is most frequently seen before 24 weeks gestation [15,16] and invariably resolves by 34 weeks gestation [31].

Ventriculomegaly is the most sensitive indicator of maldevelopment of the fetal brain and spinal cord [41], and is associated with a high fetal morbidity and mortality [26,42–44]. Ventriculomegaly is seen in up to 70% to 90% of cases of spina bifida [2,15,30]. Myelomeningocele is the most common cause of hydrocephalus in the fetus, the hydrocephalus resulting from the Chiari II malformation [45]. The ventricles are measured at the ventricular atrium, in the transverse plane, across the most posterior aspect of the glomus of the choroid plexus. The measurement is obtained perpendicular to the long axis of the ventricle, and the cursors are placed at the junction of the ventricular wall with the lumen [46]. The measurement for a normal ventricle is less than or equal to 10 mm (Fig. 9) [47].

In general, if a normal ventricular atrium and a normal cisterna magna are seen, then 95% of fetal central nervous system (CNS) anomalies can be excluded [41]. Using a transabdominal approach, the ventricular atrium can be seen 99% of the time and the cisterna magna 90% of the time on sonography [41]. When transabdominal visualization is poor, transvaginal imaging may be helpful, particularly in the late second and third trimesters [48]. In spina bifida, the prevalence of ventriculomegaly increases with increasing gestational age and with worsening posterior fossa deformity [49]. Thus, before 24 weeks gestation, the lack of ventriculomegaly should not deter one from considering the possibility of spina bifida. The degree of ventriculomegaly and the severity of posterior fossa deformity have no relation to the level of the spinal defect [50].

Other cranial findings associated with spina bifida are a small BPD for gestational age [16,35] and a small TCD. In the second trimester of normal fetuses, the TCD has been shown to correspond

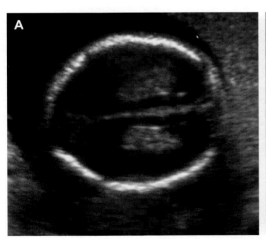
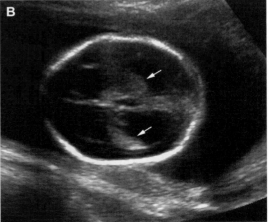

Fig. 9. Transverse views of the head in two fetuses at 18 weeks gestation. (A) Normal-sized ventricles. Note that the choroids plexus fills most of space in the lateral ventricles. (B) Both lateral ventricles are enlarged, with "dangling" choroid plexus (*arrows*).

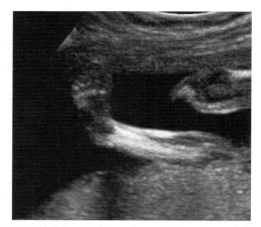

Fig. 10. Club foot at 20 weeks gestation. Coronal view shows a club foot deformity. The tibia and fibula, and the foot are seen in the long axis.

approximately to the gestational age in weeks [51]. One study of 261 fetuses with spina bifida showed that, using a TCD cutoff of less than or equal to 0.9 multiples of the median, 80% of open spina bifida could be detected, with a false-positive rate of 4% [34].

Other associated findings of spinal neural tube defects

Other CNS anomalies associated with spina bifida include holoprosencephaly, agenesis of the corpus callosum, dandy walker malformation, tethered cord, diastematomyelia, intraspinal lipoma, and dermoid cysts [52]. Other associated non-CNS anomalies include those involving the kidneys, gastrointestinal tract, face, thorax, and extremities. Fetal movements frequently appear normal, even those of the lower extremities, although at times a clubfoot deformity is present (Fig. 10).

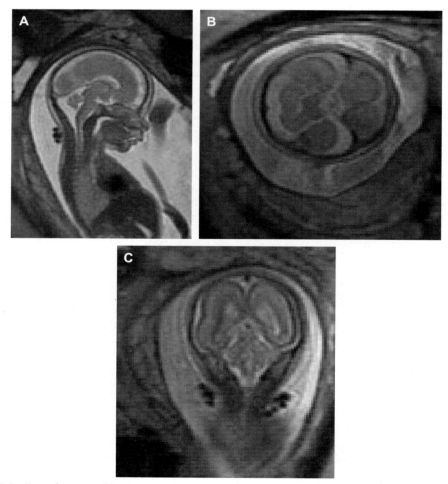

Fig. 11. MR images of a normal brain at 21 weeks gestation. Sagittal (*A*), transverse (*B*), and coronal (*C*) views show a normal appearance to the cerebellum and cisterna magna.

Multiple factors contribute to the prognosis of fetuses with spina bifida, in terms of degree of handicap and chance of survival [53]. The most important factor is the level of the lesion, with a lower spinal lesion having a better prognosis [2,54,55]. Sonographically determined levels are in agreement with the pathologic levels in 64% of cases, and are within one spinal level in 79% [56]. Factors that interfere with accurate determination of spinal level include multiple gestations, severe angulation of the spine, and the presence of other fetal anomalies [56]. The presence and degree of ventriculomegaly is a poor prognostic indicator [57,58]. The possibility for ambulation is much more likely with sacral lesions, compared with higher spinal lesions [59]; however, the movement seen in utero cannot be used to predict the level of motor function after birth [60].

MR imaging of spinal neural tube defects

Fetal MR imaging has been shown to be helpful in the evaluation of CNS anomalies [61,62]. Currently, no evidence suggests that a short-term exposure to electromagnetic fields is harmful to the fetus [63–65]. Early fetal studies were limited by motion [66–68]. Attempts to limit fetal motion included fetal umbilical vein injection of pancuronium bromide [69] and maternal sedation with benzodiazepines [70]. At the authors' institution, they use a half-Fourier single-shot rapid acquisition and relaxation enhancement technique, which limits artifacts from maternal and fetal motion because each image is obtained in about 420 milliseconds [61,71]. The normal cerebellum and cisterna magna are well depicted in the sagittal, axial, and coronal planes on MR imaging (Fig. 11). Although Chiari II malformations (Fig. 12) and spinal defects

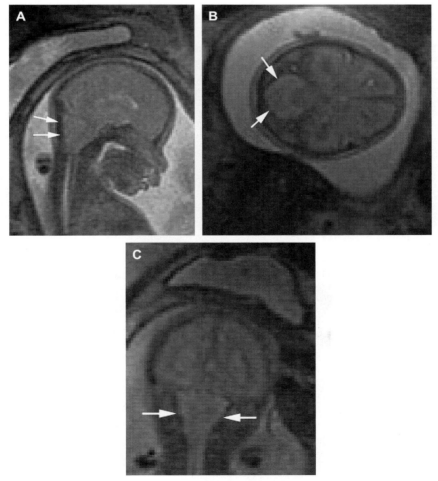

Fig. 12. MR image of fetus with Chiari II malformation. Sagittal (*A*), transverse (*B*) and coronal (*C*) views show downward herniation of the cerebellum with effacement of the cisterna magna (*arrows*).

(Fig. 13) are seen with MR imaging, small myelo-meningoceles may be difficult to see on MR images because of partial volume averaging of the thin wall of the sac surrounded by fluid on T2-weighted images [61]. On the other hand, MR may detect a caudal (low sacral) defect, which is difficult to visualize sonographically, as was the case in 1 of 16 spinal NTDs in a series by Levine and colleagues [72]; however, the intracranial findings on ultrasound did suggest the diagnosis.

In patients undergoing fetal surgery for NTDs, MR imaging can be helpful to follow the improvement in degree of herniation of the posterior fossa structures after surgery because this modality gives a better assessment of the degree of posterior fossa herniation [73].

The MR imaging appearance of the fetal cerebral ventricles in NTDs has also been reported [74]. The ventricles in cases of spinal NTD frequently have an angular configuration, a feature more likely to be present in cases with no ventriculomegaly, although it has also been seen in cases of mild to moderate ventriculomegaly (Fig. 14). This study, which reviewed the ventricular morphology in many CNS anomalies, found this appearance to be present only in cases of NTDs.

In general, however, when the myelomeningocele is well seen on sonography, and when fetal surgery is not contemplated, MR imaging has a limited role in regards to changing patient management.

Anencephaly

Anencephaly is a universally fatal type of NTD. Female fetuses are affected four times as often as male fetuses. Although anencephaly means "no brain," some abnormal brain tissue or angiomatous stroma can be present, especially in the first trimester. When a moderate amount of tissue is seen superior to the orbits, it is termed exencephaly (Fig. 15). In the first trimester, the diagnosis of anencephaly is made when the cranium and cerebral hemispheres superior to the orbits are absent. The base of the skull and orbits are nearly always present, and the brainstem and cerebellum may be spared. By the midsecond trimester, the angiomatous stroma

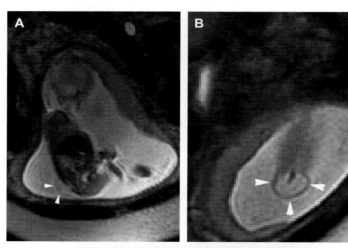

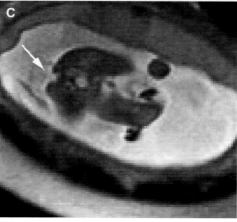

Fig. 13. Sagittal (*A*), coronal (*B*), and axial (*C*) MR images of a fetus with lumbar spine NTD at 18 weeks gestation. Note that the thin sac (*arrowheads*) is seen better on the coronal and sagittal images than on the axial image because of partial volume averaging. The axial image shows a defect in the soft tissues (*arrow*), which can aid in diagnosis when the sac is not well visualized.

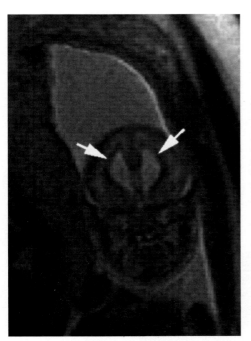

Fig. 14. Coronal MR image of a fetus with mild ventriculomegaly and NTD at 20 weeks gestation shows an angular shape to the lateral cerebral ventricles (*arrows*).

has sloughed off into the amniotic fluid, and the sonographic appearance is that of a "bug-eye," with no tissue or cranium visualized above the orbits (Fig. 16).

Polyhydramnios is a common associated finding in fetuses with anencephaly [75], but typically does not develop until the late second trimester, caused by a defect in the swallowing mechanism.

Associated CNS anomalies include spina bifida. Associated non-CNS anomalies include urinary tract anomalies (usually hydronephrosis), diaphragmatic hernia, cleft lip or palate, cardiovascular abnormalities, and gastrointestinal abnormalities including omphalocele [76].

The two main differential diagnoses include severe microcephaly and amniotic band syndrome involving the cranium. The main feature to distinguish severe microcephaly from anencephaly is the presence of the cranial vault in microcephaly. In amniotic band syndrome, the cranial defect is usually asymmetric, and other typically associated findings include limb amputation [75]. Also, amniotic band syndrome may be associated with oligohydramnios, which is uncommon in anencephaly.

Because the sonographic features of anencephaly are fairly characteristic, and because all cases are lethal, the role of MR imaging in these cases is limited.

Cephaloceles

A cephalocele is present when there is a herniation of meninges (meningocele) or brain and meninges (encephalocele) through a bony defect in the calvarium. The location of the defect can vary. The proportion of anterior and posterior defects is related to ethnicity, with the frontal defects being more common in the Eastern world and the occipital defects being more common (75%) in the Western world (Fig. 17) [77].

MSAFP is used to screen for these defects despite the fact that they are covered by skin, and thus, alpha-fetoprotein should not leak into the amniotic fluid [78]. Some hypothesize that the skin is thin and parchment-like, and may have tiny focal

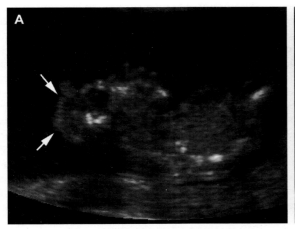

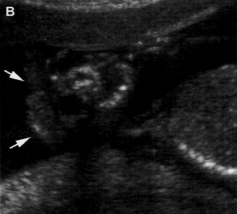

Fig. 15. Exencephaly. Sagittal (*A*) and coronal (*B*) views of a fetus at 15 weeks gestation show absence of a cranium with abnormal tissue superior to the orbits (*arrows*). This tissue will "melt" away during gestation, eventually leading to the appearance of anencephaly.

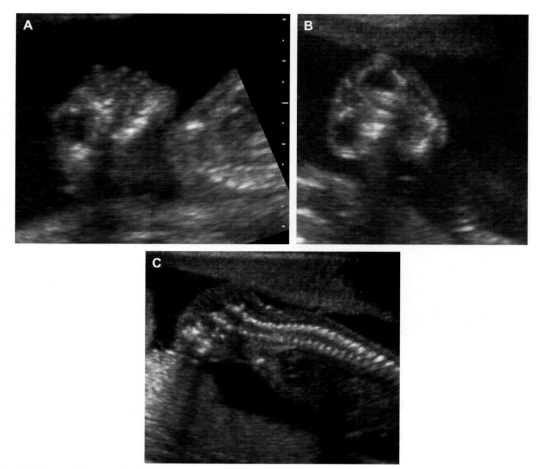

Fig. 16. Anencephaly. Sagittal (*A*) and coronal (*B, C*) views of a fetus at 18 weeks gestation show lack of tissue superior to the orbits. Note that the coronal view of the cervical spine shows splaying of the posterior elements, with the bony elements terminating at the expected location of the calvarium.

defects, thus allowing alpha-fetoprotein to leak into the amniotic fluid [79]. The MSAFP level and the size of the cephalocele are not correlated [80].

To make the diagnosis of a cephalocele on sonography, a cranial defect must be present. Care should be taken to demonstrate that the defect is real and not refraction artifact from imaging the edge of the skull tangentially. The defect, even when present, is reportedly seen with ultrasound in 80% to 96% of cases [78,80]. Thus, other extracranial masses, such as cystic hygromas, teratomas, hemangiomas, cephalohematomas, epidermal scalp cysts, and scalp edema, can mimic cephaloceles if care is not taken to assess the underlying cranial defect.

An important prognostic indicator is the presence of neural tissue in the herniated sac, because meningoceles have a better prognosis than encephaloceles [81]. Frontal cephaloceles have a better prognosis than occipital cephaloceles [82]. Other

prognostic indicators include the size of the lesion, the amount of brain tissue present in the sac, ventriculomegaly, microcephaly, and associated anomalies [77].

In one study, 44% of fetuses with cephalocele had associated abnormal karyotypes [78]. Syndromes can also be associated, including Meckel-Gruber, which is an autosomal recessive disorder with occipital encephalocele, bilateral cystic kidneys (with the appearance of autosomal recessive polycystic kidney disease), and postaxial polydactyly. In general, the overall survival is poor for encephalocele, reported at 21% to 22% for in utero series [78,80] and 50% to 56% for pediatric series [83,84]. Most of these patients have significant developmental delay and neurologic impairment.

MR imaging of cephaloceles

Ultrasound cannot always differentiate meningoceles from encephaloceles [78,81]. MR imaging plays a critical role in characterizing the contents of the herniated sac and assessing the intracranial anatomy, findings that have a critical role in diagnosis, counseling, management, and prognosis (Figs. 17 and 18) [85,86]. In cases of encephalocele, MR imaging can show the underlying brain to appear normal (see Fig. 18A) or abnormal (see Fig. 18B). In some cases, because of fetal position, the encephalocele itself may be difficult to visualize with ultrasound, but is better seen with MR imaging (see Fig. 18C). The additional information provided by MR imaging can help identify cases with more favorable prognosis and cases with poor prognosis. Even when ultrasound shows the findings well, MR imaging is helpful for the patients and the neurologists counseling the patients in terms of better visualizing and understanding the anomalies present.

Summary

Myelomeningoceles

- Myelomeningocele is seen on ultrasound as a defect in the spine, usually the lumbosacral spine, with a protruding cystic lesion containing neural elements.
- Even when a spinal defect is not seen, the diagnosis should be suspected when the cranial abnormalities associated with Chiari II malformation are present.
- Most important prognostic factor is the level of the spinal defect.
- An angular appearance to the ventricles is highly specific for NTD.
- MR imaging has a limited role, except for cases in which fetal surgery is contemplated.

Anencephaly

- Diagnosis can be made in the first trimester.
- Characteristic appearance is absence of cranium and cerebral hemispheres above the orbits.

Cephaloceles

- Fetus must have a cranial defect to make this diagnosis.
- Cephaloceles can contain meninges or brain and meninges (encephalocele).

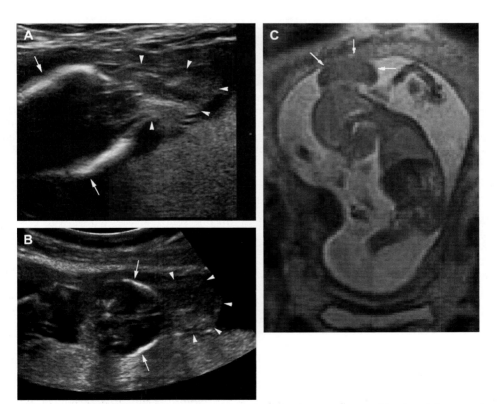

Fig. 17. Fetus at 17 weeks gestation. Axial (*A*) and coronal (*B*) ultrasound images of the head show an abnormal skull (*large arrows*) with a large defect with a large amount of extracranial material (*arrowheads*). (*C*) Sagittal MR image shows the lack of normal brain structures, with large encephalocele (*small arrows*).

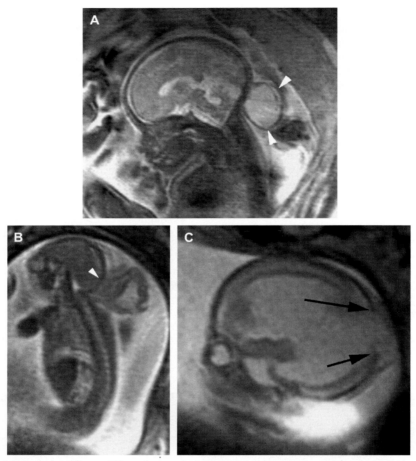

Fig. 18. Three MR images of three different second trimester fetuses with encephaloceles. (*A*) Note the sac with only a small amount of tissue (*arrowheads*) and otherwise normal-appearing intracranial anatomy. (*B*) Note the large amount of tissue in the sac (*arrowhead*) and the sloping forehead appearance of microcephaly. (*C*) Note the large posterior defect (*arrows*) and ventriculomegaly. (*Reproduced from* Levine D, Barnes P. MR imaging of fetal CNS abnormalities. In: Levine D, editor. Atlas of fetal MRI. 1st edition. Boca Raton (FL): Taylor & Francis Group; 2005. p. 34–5; with permission.)

- Occipital location is the most common in Western world.
- MR imaging plays a critical role in assessing the underlying intracranial anatomy, findings that determine prognosis.

References

[1] Greenberg F, James LM, Oakley GP Jr. Estimates of birth prevalence rates of spina bifida in the United States from computer generated maps. Am J Obstet Gynecol 1983;145(5):570–3.

[2] Main DM, Mennuti MT. Neural tube defects: issues in prenatal diagnosis and counseling. Obstet Gynecol 1986;67(1):1–16.

[3] Drugan A, Johnson MP, Dvorin E, et al. Aneuploidy with neural tube defects: another reason for complete evaluation in patients with suspected ultrasound anomalies or elevated maternal serum alpha-fetoprotein. Fetal Ther 1989;4(2–3):88–92.

[4] Chung CS, Myrianthopoulos NC. Racial and prenatal factors in major congenital malformations. Am J Hum Genet 1968;20(1):44–60.

[5] Lemire RJ. Neural tube defects. JAMA 1988; 259(4):558–62.

[6] Kennedy D, Chitayat D, Winsor EJT, et al. Prenatally diagnosed neural tube defects: ultrasound, chromosome and autopsy or postnatal findings in 212 cases. Am J Med Genet 1998;77(4):317–21.

[7] Vogel F, Motulsky AG. Human genetics. 3rd edition. New York: Springer-Verlag; 1996. 210–6.

[8] Holmes LB, Driscoll SG, Atkins L. Etiologic heterogeneity of neural tube defects. N Engl J Med 1976;294(7):365–9.

[9] Khoury MJ, Erickson JD, James LM. Etiologic heterogeneity of neural tube defects: clues from epidemiology. Am J Epidemiol 1982;115(4): 538–48.

[10] Khoury MJ, Erickson JD, James LM. Etiologic heterogeneity of neural tube defects II: clues from family studies. Am J Hum Genet 1982; 34(6):980–7.

[11] Robert E, Guibaud P. Maternal valproic acid and congenital neural tube defects. Lancet 1982; 2(8304):937.

[12] Jones KL, Lacro RV, Johnson KA, et al. Pattern of malformations in children of women treated with carbamazepine during pregnancy. N Engl J Med 1989;320(25):1661–6.

[13] Harmon JP, Hiett AK, Palmer CG, et al. Prenatal ultrasound detection of isolated neural tube defects: is cytogenetic evaluation warranted? Obstet Gynecol 1995;86(1 Pt 1):595–9.

[14] Luthy DA, Wardinsky T, Shurleff DB, et al. Cesarean section before onset of labor and subsequent motor function in infants with meningomyelocele diagnosed antenatally. N Engl J Med 1991; 324(10):662–6.

[15] Watson WJ, Chescheir NC, Katz VL, et al. The role of ultrasound in evaluation of patients with elevated maternal serum alpha-fetoprotein: a review. Obstet Gynecol 1991;78(1):123–8.

[16] Van den Hof MC, Nicolaides KH, Campbell J, et al. Evaluation of the lemon and banana signs in one hundred thirty fetuses with open spina bifida. Am J Obstet Gynecol 1990;162(2): 322–7.

[17] Morrow RJ, McNay MB, Whittle NJ. Ultrasound detection of neural tube defects in patients with elevated maternal serum alpha-fetoprotein. Obstet Gynecol 1991;78(6):1055–7.

[18] Shields LE, Uhrich SB, Komarniski CA, et al. Amniotic fluid alpha-fetoprotein determination at the time of genetic amniocentesis: has it outlived its usefulness? J Ultrasound Med 1996; 15(11):735–9.

[19] Campbell J, Gilbert WM, Nicolaides KH, et al. Ultrasound screening for spina bifida: cranial and cerebellar signs in a high risk population. Obstet Gynecol 1987;70(2):247–50.

[20] American Institute of Ultrasound in Medicine. AIUM practice guidelines for the performance of an antepartum obstetric ultrasound examination. Laurel (MD). American Institute of Ultrasound in Medicine 2003. Available at: http://www.aium.org/publications/clinical/obstetrical.pdf. Accessed February 15, 2007.

[21] Filly RA, Golbus MS. Ultrasonography of the normal and pathologic fetal skeleton. Radiol Clin North Am 1982;20(2):311–23.

[22] Filly RA, Simpson GF, Linkowski G. Fetal spine morphology and maturation during the second trimester. J Ultrasound Med 1987;6(1):631–6.

[23] Budorick NE, Pretorius DH, Grafe MR, et al. Ossification of the fetal spine. Radiology 1991; 181(2):561–5.

[24] Dennis MA, Drose JA, Pretorius DH, et al. Normal fetal sacrum simulating spina bifida: "pseudodysraphism". Radiology 1985;155(3):751–4.

[25] Harrison LA, Pretorius DH, Budorick NE. Abnormal spinal curvature in the fetus. J Ultrasound Med 1992;11(9):473–9.

[26] Nicolaides KH, Campbell S, Gabbe SG, et al. Ultrasound screening for spina bifida: cranial and cerebellar signs. Lancet 1986;2(8498):72–4.

[27] Nyberg DA, Mack LA, Hirsh J, et al. Fetal hydrocephalus: sonographic detection and clinical significance of associated anomalies. Radiology 1987;163(1):187–91.

[28] Benacerraf BR, Stryker J, Frigoletto FD. Abnormal US appearance of the cerebellum (banana sign): indirect sign of spina bifida. Radiology 1989;171(1):151–3.

[29] Pilu G, Romero R, Reece EA, et al. Subnormal cerebellum in fetuses with spina bifida. Am J Obstet Gynecol 1988;158(5):1052–6.

[30] Goldstein RB, Podrasky AE, Filly RA, et al. Effacement of the fetal cisterna magna in association with myelomeningocele. Radiology 1989; 172(2):409–13.

[31] Nyberg DA, Mack LA, Hirsch J, et al. Abnormalities of the fetal cranial contour in sonographic detection of spina bifida: evaluation of the "lemon" sign. Radiology 1988;167(2): 387–92.

[32] Penso C, Redline RW, Benacerraf BR. A sonographic sign which predicts which fetuses with hydrocephalus have an associated neural tube defect. J Ultrasound Med 1987;6(6):307–11.

[33] Furness ME, Barbary JE, Verco PW. Fetal head shape in spina bifida in the second trimester. J Clin Ultrasound 1987;15(7):451–3.

[34] De Courcy-Wheeler RH, Pomeranz MM, Wald NJ, et al. Small fetal transverse cerebellar diameter: a screening test for spina bifida. Br J Obstet Gynaecol 1994;101(10):904–5.

[35] Wald N, Cuckle H, Boreham J, et al. Small biparietal diameter of fetuses with spina bifida: implications for antenatal screening. Br J Obstet Gynaecol 1980;87(3):219–21.

[36] Mahoney BS, Callen PW, Filly RA, et al. The fetal cisterna magna. Radiology 1984;153(3):773–6.

[37] Blumenfeld Z, Siegler E, Bronshtein M. The early diagnosis of neural tube defects. Prenat Diagn 1993;13(9):863–71.

[38] McLone DG, Knepper PA. The cause of the Chiari II malformation: a unified theory. Pediatr Neurosci 1989;15(1):1–12.

[39] Ball RH, Filly RA, Goldstein RB, et al. The lemon sign: not a specific indicator of menignomyelocele. J Ultrasound Med 1993;12(3):131–4.

[40] Filly RA. The "lemon" sign: a clinical perspective. Radiology 1988;167(2):573–5.

[41] Filly RA, Cardoza JD, Goldstein RB, et al. Detection of fetal central nervous system anomalies: a

practical level of effort for a routine sonogram. Radiology 1989;172(2):403–8.

[42] Mahony BS, Nyberg DA, Hirsch JH, et al. Mild idiopathic lateral cerebral ventriculomegaly: associated anomalies and fetal outcome. Radiology 1988;169(3):715–21.

[43] Pretorius DH, Davis K, Manco-Johnson ML, et al. Clinical course of hydrocephalus: 40 cases. AJR Am J Roentgenol 1985;144(4):827–31.

[44] Hudgins RJ, Edwards MS, Goldstein R, et al. Natural history of fetal ventriculomegaly. Pediatrics 1988;82(5):692–7.

[45] Filly RA. Ultrasound evaluation of the fetal neural axis. In: Callen PW, editor. Ultrasonography in obstetrics and gynecology. Pennsylvania (PA): WB Saunders Company; 1994. p. 228.

[46] Heiserman J, Filly RA, Goldstein RB. Effect of measurement errors on sonographic evaluation of ventriculomegaly. J Ultrasound Med 1991; 10(3):121–4.

[47] Cardoza JD, Goldstein RB, Filly RA. Exclusion of fetal ventriculomegaly with a single measurement: the width of the lateral ventricular atrium. Radiology 1988;169(3):711–4.

[48] Montaegudo A, Ruess ML, Timor-Tritsch IE. Imaging the fetal brain in the second and third trimesters using transvaginal sonography. Obstet Gynecol 1991;77(1):27–32.

[49] Babcock CJ, Goldstein RB, Barth RA, et al. Prevalence of ventriculomegaly in association with myelomeningocele: correlation with gestational age and severity of posterior fossa deformity. Radiology 1994;190(3):703–7.

[50] Babcock CJ, Drake CM, Goldstein RB. Spinal level of fetal myelomeningocele: does it influence ventricular size? AJR 1997;169(1):207–10.

[51] Goldstein I, Reece EA, Pilu G, et al. Cerebellar measurements with ultrasonography in the evaluation of fetal growth and development. Am J Obstet Gynecol 1987;156(5):1065–9.

[52] Nyberg DA, Mach LA. The spine and neural tube defects. St Louis (MO): Mosby Yearbook; 1990.

[53] Laurence KM. Effect of early surgery for spina bifida cystica on survival and quality of life. Lancet 1974;1(7852):301–4.

[54] Ames MD, Schut L. Results of treatment of 171 consecutive myelomeningoceles: 1963 to 1968. Pediatrics 1972;50(3):466–70.

[55] Kupka J, Geddes N, Carroll NC. Comprehensive management in the child with spina bifida. Orthop Clin North Am 1978;9(1):97–113.

[56] Kollias SS, Goldstein RB, Cogen PH, et al. Prenatally detected myelomeningoceles: sonographic accuracy in estimation of the spinal level. Radiology 1992;185(1):109–12.

[57] Coniglio SJ, Anderson SM, Ferguson JE. Developmental outcomes of children with myelomeningocele: prenatal predictors. Am J Obstet Gynecol 1997;177(2):319–26.

[58] Mapstone TB, Rekate HL, Nulsen PF, et al. Relationship of SCF shunting and IQ in children

with myelomeningocele: a retrospective analysis. Child's Brain 1984;11(2):112–8.

[59] Cochrane DD, Wilson RD, Steinbok P, et al. Prenatal spinal evaluation and functional outcome of patients born with myelomeningocele: information for improved prenatal counseling and outcome prediction. Fetal Diagn Ther 1996; 11(3):159–68.

[60] Warsof SL, Abramowicz JS, Sayegh SK, et al. Lower limb movements and urologic function in fetuses with neural tube and other central nervous system defects. Fetal Ther 1988;3(3):129–34.

[61] Levine D, Barnes PD, Madsen JR, et al. Fetal central nervous system anomalies: MR imaging augments sonographic diagnosis. Radiology 1997;204(3):635–42.

[62] Yuh WT, Nyugen HD, Fisher DJ, et al. MR of fetal central nervous system abnormalities. AJNR Am J Neuroradiol 1994;15(3):459–64.

[63] Baker P, Johnson I, Harvey P, et al. Three-year follow up of children imaged in utero using echo planar magnetic resonance. Am J Obstet Gynecol 1994;170(1 Pt 1):32–3.

[64] Kanal E, Gillen J, Evans J, et al. Survey of reproductive health among female MR workers. Radiology 1993;187(2):395–9.

[65] Reid A, Smith F, Hutchinson J. Nuclear magnetic resonance imaging and its safety implications: follow up of 181 patients. Br J Radiol 1982; 55(658):784–6.

[66] McCarthy SM, Filly RA, Stark DD, et al. Magnetic resonance imaging of fetal anomalies in utero: early experience. AJR Am J Roentgenol 1985; 145(4):677–82.

[67] Johnson IR, Symonds EM, Kean DM, et al. Imaging the pregnant human uterus with nuclear magnetic resonance. Am J Obstet Gynecol 1984;148(8):1136–9.

[68] Stark D, McCarthy S, Filly RA, et al. Intrauterine growth retardation: evaluation by magnetic resonance—work in progress. Radiology 1985; 155(2):425–7.

[69] Williamson RA, Weiner CP, Yuh WT, et al. Magnetic resonance imaging of anomalous fetuses. Obstet Gynecol 1989;73(6):952–6.

[70] Weinreb JC, Lowe TW, Santos-Ramos R, et al. Magnetic resonance imaging in obstetric diagnosis. Radiology 1985;154(1):157–61.

[71] Levine D, Hatabu H, Gaa J, et al. Fetal anatomy revealed with fast MR sequences. AJR Am J Roentgenol 1996;167(4):905–8.

[72] Levine D. MR imaging of fetal central nervous system abnormalities. Brain Cogn 2002;50(3): 432–48.

[73] Sutton LN, Adzick NS, Bilaniuk LT, et al. Improvement in hindbrain herniation demonstrated by serial fetal magnetic resonance imaging following fetal surgery for myelomeningocele. JAMA 1999;282(19):1826–31.

[74] Levine D, Trop I, Mehta TS, et al. MR imaging appearance of fetal cerebral ventricular morphology. Radiology 2002;223(3):652–60.

[75] Goldstein RB, Filly RA. Prenatal diagnosis of anencephaly: spectrum of sonographic appearances and distinction from the amniotic band syndrome. AJR Am J Roentgenol 1988;151(3): 547–50.

[76] David TJ, Nixon A. Congenital malformations associated with anencephaly and iniencephaly. J Med Genet 1976;13(4):263–5.

[77] Hanley ML, Guzman ER, Vintzileos AM, et al. Prenatal ultrasonographic detection of regression of an encephalocele. J Ultrasound Med 1996;15(1):71–4.

[78] Goldstein RB, LaPidus AS, Filly RA. Fetal cephaloceles: diagnosis with US. Radiology 1991; 180(3):803–8.

[79] Naidich TP, Altman NR, Braffman BH, et al. Cephaloceles and related malformations. AJNR 1992;13(2):655–90.

[80] Budorick NE, Pretorius DH, McGahan JP, et al. Cephalocele detection in utero: sonographic and clinical features. Ultrasound Obstet Gynecol 1995;5(2):77–85.

[81] Chervenak FA, Isaacson G, Mahoney MJ, et al. Diagnosis and management of fetal cephalocele. Obstet Gynecol 1984;64(1):86–91.

[82] French BN. Midline fusion defects and defects of formation. In: Youmans JR, editor. 3rd edition. Neurological surgery, vol. 2. Philadelphia: Saunders; 1990. p. 1150–235.

[83] Lorber J. The prognosis of occipital encephalocele. Dev Med Child Neurol 1967;(Suppl) 13:75–86.

[84] Mealey J, Dzenitis AJ, Hockey AA. The prognosis of encephaloceles. J Neurosurg 1970;32(2):209–18.

[85] Levine D, Barnes PD, Robertson RR, et al. Fast MR imaging of fetal central nervous system abnormalities. Radiology 2003;229(1):51–61.

[86] Levine D, Barnes P. MR imaging of fetal CNS abnormalities. In: Levine D, editor. Atlas of fetal MRI. 1st edition. Boca Raton (FL): Taylor & Francis Group; 2005. p. 25–72.

ULTRASOUND
CLINICS

Ultrasound Clin 2 (2007) 203–215

ELSEVIER
SAUNDERS

Quantitative Approaches for Volume Sonography During Pregnancy

Wesley Lee, MD, FACOG, FAIUM[a,b,*]

- ▪ Technical considerations
- ▪ Quantitative analysis of volume data
  Spina bifida
  Characterization of jaw development
  Micrognathia/retrognathia Volume
    measurements

- *Tissue perfusion*
  Detection of Down syndrome
- ▪ Summary
- ▪ References

As three-dimensional ultrasound imaging technology becomes more widely available, health care providers should understand how software tools can be used to evaluate suspected fetal anomalies. In 2005, the American Institute of Ultrasound in Medicine sponsored a Consensus Conference to provide guidance on this matter [1]. Volume sonography was described as a complementary imaging technology that has "added diagnostic and clinical value for selected indications and circumstances in obstetric and gynecologic ultrasound." The importance of standardized views and postprocessing techniques was also emphasized.

A companion article in the same issue of the *Journal of Ultrasound in Medicine* reviewed available literature regarding how this technology was being used in obstetric practice [2]. Specific clinical benefit was found for diagnostic problems that included facial anomalies, neural tube defects, and skeletal malformations. Other potential areas of benefit included the prenatal diagnosis of congenital heart disease, fetal weight estimation and growth assessment, improvement of clinical efficiency, parental bonding, remote diagnosis, medical education, and training. Despite current emphasis on the qualitative evaluation of multiplanar and surface-rendered images, other important tools can be used during pregnancy. This article reviews basic approaches for the quantitative analysis of selected fetal abnormalities that are encountered during clinical practice.

Technical considerations

Conventional ultrasound systems create images based on sound waves that propagate through biologic tissue. High-frequency sound waves are reflected by boundaries between tissue or fluid interfaces. More than 4 decades ago, an engineer from the Jet Propulsion Laboratory described the smallest picture elements of video images from space probes as being a picture element or "pixel" [3,4]. Square or rectangular pixels are composed of data bits that contain gray-scale or color-depth information for each image. For example, one pixel contains 2^8 intensity values for "8-bit gray scale" or 2^{24} (ie, 6,777,216 colors) for "24-bit color" images.

Three-dimensional ultrasonography (3DUS) is based on volume-based pixels or "voxel" elements, which allow the visualization of fetal structures. Each voxel has known geometric and physical

[a] Division of Fetal Imaging, William Beaumont Hospital, 3601 West Thirteen Mile Road, Royal Oak, MI 48073-6769, USA
[b] Department of Obstetrics and Gynecology, Wayne State University, Detroit, MI, USA
* Division of Fetal Imaging, William Beaumont Hospital, 3601 West Thirteen Mile Road, Royal Oak, MI 48073-6769.
E-mail address: wlee@beaumont.edu

1556-858X/07/$ – see front matter © 2007 Elsevier Inc. All rights reserved.
ultrasound.theclinics.com

doi:10.1016/j.cult.2007.07.004

dimensions that make accurate volume calculations possible. They are specified by their location in three-dimensional (3D) space and may contain additional information regarding opacity, transparency, and gray-scale or color intensity values.

Some general guidelines should be considered for optimal acquisition of satisfactory volume data. First, the examiner must decide which volume analysis tools are best suited to address a specific clinical problem. In some situations, 3DUS is not likely to offer additional insight over the initial diagnostic impression given by conventional sonography. Second, the best quality 3D volume datasets result from optimizing two-dimensional images during data acquisition. For example, the original ultrasound images should be magnified adequately to fill most of the display screen, the focal zone should be centered on the anatomic region of interest, and the system gain should be adjusted appropriately. Third, other factors, such as maternal wall thickness, amniotic fluid volume, fetal size, and fetal position, should be considered before deciding how best to acquire this volume data.

Quantitative analysis of volume data

Many common problems encountered during clinical practice can be identified and well characterized by two-dimensional ultrasonography (2DUS). Occasionally, the initial diagnostic impression is not made confidently or questions may linger about the nature of the finding. Under these circumstances, one should weigh the potential benefits for using one of several different volume analysis tools for answering specific diagnostic questions. Volume datasets can be explored further using various commercially available software packages (eg, 4D View, GE Healthcare; Q-Lab, Philips Medical Systems; SonoView Pro, Medison; *four*Sight View-Tool, Siemens Medical Solutions). Despite similar capabilities, this article emphasizes quantitative approaches using 4D View software for demonstration purposes.

Spina bifida

Background

The prenatal diagnosis of spina bifida has improved steadily as a result of maternal serum alpha-fetoprotein screening and the widespread use of ultrasonography. Corresponding advances in patient management have greatly reduced mortality, but have had minimal impact on long-term disability from neurologic sequelae. This morbidity includes paraplegia, sensory deficits, spinal deformity, bowel dysfunction, and urinary incontinence.

Prenatal ultrasonography can detect many fetuses with spina bifida and this information is commonly used to determine the extent of a spinal lesion for prognostic significance. Kollias and colleagues [5] reported that 2DUS estimated the defect to within one vertebral segment in 79% of fetuses with spina bifida. One retrospective study of 171 consecutive cases of spina bifida, however, found that only 29% of cases accurately identified the specific upper level of a spinal lesion [6]. Other investigators have suggested that 3DUS may further characterize spina bifida [7–10].

Technique

A semiquantitative technique has been described as a standardized approach for determining the anatomic level of spina bifida (Fig. 1A–C) [11]. Multiplanar views are acquired using a volume probe from an axial sweep of the fetal spine. A coronal view of the lumbar and sacral spine is rendered with a maximum intensity projection algorithm that primarily displays the bony spine. An electronic cutting plane is used to display orthogonal views of the volume-rendered spine, beginning at the spinal segment that is contiguous with the last fetal rib. As the examiner moves the cutting plane toward the sacral spine, simultaneous views of the axial spine and over-lying skin line can be visualized.

Important points

- Accurate characterization of spina bifida relies on sonographic recognition of disrupted ossification centers or overlying skin from transverse and coronal views of the fetal spine.
- Sonography predicts the clinical severity of open spina bifida because neurologic symptoms correlate with the anatomic level of the defect.
- Three-dimensional ultrasonography provides useful multiplanar views for the evaluation of spina bifida. Optimal views can be generated by manipulation of a virtual cutting plane through a volume reconstruction of the fetal spine.
- Spinal defect levels obtained in this manner closely correlate with findings from 2DUS and postnatal results. However, it may be prudent to count the total number of ribs carefully to assume correctly that the last rib correctly corresponds to the twelfth thoracic vertebra.
- Although multiplanar views are generally more informative than rendered views for localizing these defects, their simultaneous use increases the likelihood that a spinal defect will be appropriately analyzed.

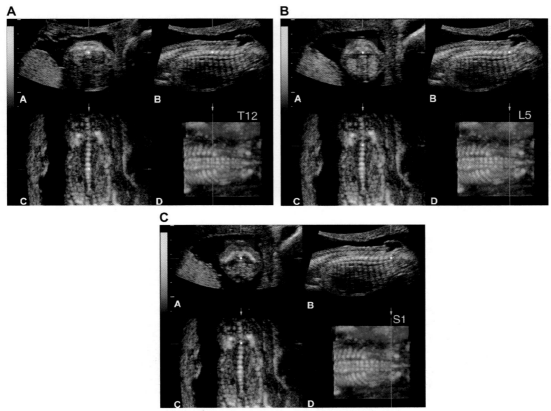

Fig. 1. (*A*) Multiplanar view of spina bifida. A common reference dot represents the same spatial coordinate within the volume data from intersecting orthogonal planes. Window A (*top left*) represents the original axial plane of data acquisition. A "region of interest" is accepted, using a light rectangular box that includes the spine with overlying skin line. Window B (*top right*) results from a midline sagittal cutting plane from Window A. Window C is a coronal reconstruction of the orange horizontal cutting plane seen in Window A. Window D displays a rendered spine, using a maximum intensity projection filter that primarily displays echogenic bone. A green vertical line is manually placed on the 12th thoracic vertebra with the last fetal rib. The examiner can simultaneously visualize the intact posterior ossification elements and overlying skin line from an axial view of the spine (*Window A*). (*Reproduced from* Lee W, Chaiworapongsa T, Romero R, et al. A diagnostic approach for the evaluation of spina bifida by three-dimensional ultrasonography. J Ultrasound Med 2002;21:619–26; with permission.) (*B*) Sequential analysis of spinal segments. The green cutting line is manually moved along each spinal segment toward the sacrum. At the L5 level, an axial view of the overlying spinal skin demonstrates some thickening (*Window A*). (*C*) Semiquantitative localization of an upper spinal defect. At the level of the first sacral vertebrae (S1), an axial view demonstrates a disruption of posterior spinal elements and overlying skin (*Window A*). By sequential analysis, the examiner has increased diagnostic confidence that the upper extent of the spinal defect is between the L5 and S1 vertebrae. (*Reproduced from* Lee W, Chaiworapongsa T, Romero R, et al. A diagnostic approach for the evaluation of spina bifida by three-dimensional ultrasonography. J Ultrasound Med 2002;21:619–26; with permission.)

This approach may improve the characterization of spina bifida by adding diagnostic information that is complementary to the initial assessment by 2DUS.

Characterization of jaw development

Background

Micrognathia refers to a facial malformation that results from a small chin, whereas retrognathia is defined by posterior displacement of the mandible. The Online Mendelian Inheritance in Man database at the National Library of Medicine describes more than 299 genetic conditions that are associated with micrognathia and 47 syndromes that include retrognathia [12].

Affected fetuses with abnormal development of the maxilla or mandible are at increased risk for having a genetic syndrome. An underdeveloped chin may even be severe enough to cause hydramnios in the fetus, or respiratory obstruction after delivery. Furthermore, its presence may complicate infant feeding and typically requires one or more reparative surgeries [13].

Three-dimensional multiplanar views can be used to display true orthogonal scanning planes of the head, including a midline sagittal view of the facial profile to improve diagnostic confidence regarding the possibility of jaw anomalies [14]. It may be important to distinguish between micrognathia and retrognathia. Wulfsberg and colleagues [15] have described retrognathia with a normal-sized mandible in cases of deletion 22q11.2 syndrome, occurring because the cranial base angle is larger than normal [16]. Until recently, precise methods for the prenatal diagnosis of these anomalies have not been available.

Technique

Rotten and colleagues [17] have developed a standardized approach to the prenatal diagnosis of retrognathia and micrognathia, using 3DUS. They studied normal fetuses to establish nomograms for these anomalies.

Retrognathia   The inferior facial angle was defined from a sagittal view of the head by the intersection of two lines. The first reference line was made orthogonal to the vertical part of the forehead, drawn at the level of the synostosis of the nasal bones (Fig. 2A). A second profile line was extended from the tip of the mentum and anterior border of the more anterior lip. An inferior facial angle of less than 49.2° defined retrognathia (Fig. 2B).

Micrognathia   The mandible and maxilla width were measured on an axial view of the cranial base at the level of the maxillary and mandibular tooth buds. The mandible and maxilla widths were taken at a point that corresponded to 10 mm posterior to the anterior osseous border of the maxillary or mandibular tooth buds (Fig. 2C, D). A mandible/maxilla ratio of less than 0.0785 defined micrognathia (Fig. 2E).

Important points

 The primary value of a 3D multiplanar view is its ability to display a midline sagittal view of the fetal facial profile. This first step is important for qualitative and quantitative assessment of the fetal jaw using standardized 3DUS.
 The chin can falsely appear to be small if surrounding soft tissue is redundant (eg, macrosomia).
 Quantitative measurements of the inferior facial angle, maxilla, and mandible are helpful for

distinguishing between micrognathia and retrognathia in cases where visual assessment is questionable.

Micrognathia/retrognathia volume measurements

Three-dimensional ultrasonography makes it possible to create contiguous slices of an organ with borders that are segmented by using either manual tracing or a software-based border detection algorithm. The slice geometry is defined by known thickness and each section contains a discrete number of voxels with fixed dimensions. Studies have shown 3DUS to be more accurate than 2DUS for providing quantitative volume measurements of small irregular objects [18].

One widely used and reproducible method of volume determination using 3DUS is called VOCAL (*Virtual Organ Computer-Aided Analysis*) (Fig. 3A) [19–21]. The main advantage of this technique is that it reduces the amount of time needed to make standardized volume measurements by rotating selected slice data around a user-defined central axis. This information also allows the examiner to create surface models that are representative of volume data (Fig. 3B) [22].

Several investigators have also described 3DUS for volume measurements of the heart [23], lungs [24], placenta [25], embryo [26], gestational sac [27], and amniotic fluid [28]. The use of organ volume measurements for clinical care, however, is still an emerging concept for the diagnosis and management of fetal abnormalities. Toward this end, the authors describe in detail three areas of potential clinical benefit from fetal volume measurements for the detection of fetuses at risk for chromosomal anomalies, pulmonary hypoplasia, and fetal growth problems.

Head and trunk volume measurements and chromosomal anomalies

Falcon and colleagues [26] examined fetal head and trunk volumes in 140 chromosomally abnormal pregnancies between 11 and 13.9 weeks, menstrual age. In trisomy 21 (n = 72) and Turner syndrome (n = 14) fetuses, the crown–rump length was similar when compared with the abnormal group. However, the fetal trunk and head volumes were about 10% to 15% lower ($P<.001$ and $P = .004$, respectively). In trisomy 18 (n = 29), trisomy 13 (n = 14), and triploidy (n = 11), the deficit in volume was about 45% ($P<.001$), as compared with the deficit in crown–rump length, which was less than 15% ($P<.001$). Volume measurements of fetal head and trunk volume may improve our ability to detect growth impairment during early pregnancy in some cases of aneuploidy.

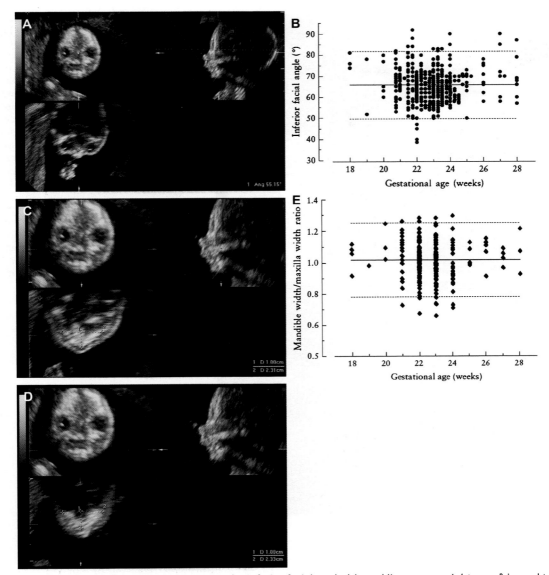

Fig. 2. (*A*) Inferior facial angle measurement. The inferior facial angle (*dotted lines, upper right panel*) is used to evaluate the possibility of retrognathia. (*B*) Value distribution of inferior facial angle as a function of gestational age in normal fetuses (measured in 371 fetuses with no known pathology.) Solid line, mean; dotted lines, ± 2 standard deviations. (*Reproduced from* Rotten D, Levaillant JM, Martinez H, et al. The fetal mandible: a 2D and 3D sonographic approach to the diagnosis of retrognathia and micrognathia. Ultrasound Obstet Gynecol 2002;19:122–30; with permission.) (*C*) Maxillary diameter measurement. An axial view (*lower left*) allows one to evaluate the maxillary alveolar tooth buds for the possibility of an anterior hard palate defect. The maxillary diameter measurement (*lower left*) is used to evaluate the fetus for micrognathia. (*D*) Mandibular diameter measurement. Similar to the maxillary diameter, the mandibular diameter measurement reflects the size of the lower jaw. A mandible-width/maxilla-width ratio of less than 0.785 defines micrognathia [17]. (*E*) Distribution of mandible-width/maxilla-width ratio as a function of gestational age in normal fetuses (measured in 245 fetuses with no known pathology). Solid line, mean; dotted lines, ± 2 standard deviations. (*Reproduced from* Rotten D, Levaillant JM, Martinez H, et al. The fetal mandible: a 2D and 3D sonographic approach to the diagnosis of retrognathia and micrognathia. Ultrasound Obstet Gynecol 2002;19:122–30; with permission.)

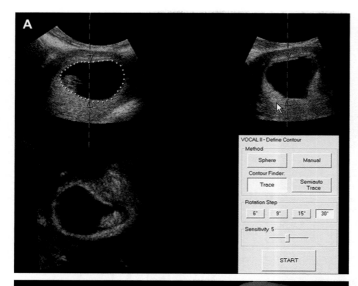

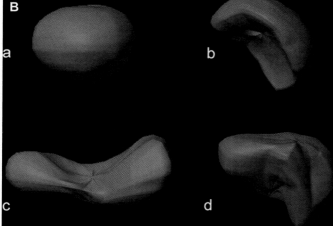

Fig. 3. (*A*) VOCAL measurement technique. Gestational sac volume can be calculated by manually rotating the gestational sac around a central axis using several user-defined steps of 6°, 9°, 15°, or 30° increments. For 30° increments, only six slices are traced. The software tool allows one to trace contours as seen above, or to apply an automated border detection algorithm by adjusting sensitivity. (*B*) Variable gestational sac shapes using the VOCAL technique. (*a*) Ellipsoid (*b*) Disk - concave (*c*) Ellipsoid - concave (*d*) Ellipsoid - irregular. (*Reproduced from* Lee W, Deter RL, McNie B, et al. Quantitative and morphological assessment of early gestational sacs using three-dimensional ultrasonography. Ultrasound Obstet Gynecol 2006;28:255–60; with permission.)

Lung volume measurements for prediction of pulmonary hypoplasia

The risk of pulmonary hypoplasia is a diagnostic challenge for fetuses that are predisposed to this condition from congenital diaphragmatic hernia. Kalache and coworkers [29] compared the use of VOCAL to a manual 3D multiplanar method for lung volume measurements among 32 fetuses at risk for pulmonary hypoplasia. Substantial agreement was observed between the results of the two approaches (95% limits of agreement were −4.4 to 8.9 mL and −3.4 to 4.8 mL, for the right and left lungs, respectively). They concluded that fetal lung volume measurements could be obtained using either method. In this study, however, the VOCAL method was associated with a lower degree of agreement and significantly higher interobserver

variability, when compared with 3D multiplanar measurements.

Another study compared the accuracy and precision of fetal lung volume measurements from VOCAL with postmortem lung volumes from water displacement [30]. The study included 8 cases of congenital diaphragmatic hernia and 25 controls without pulmonary malformation, immediately before termination. The mean relative error of lung volumes using VOCAL was −7.2% (95% confidence interval range −42.7% to +18.1%) for fetuses with congenital diaphragmatic hernia, compared with control cases (−0.7%, 95% confidence interval range −30.3% to 19.2%). Their results suggested that VOCAL is reliable for fetal lung volume estimation, even when the lungs are very small. This research group subsequently developed a nomogram of fetal lung volumes using the VOCAL technique [31].

Fractional thigh volume for fetal weight estimation

Fetal growth abnormalities are an important cause of poor neonatal outcome, but they also pose significant implications for the development of diseases in adult life. Mounting scientific evidence indicates that low birth weight can be associated with shortened lifespan and certain chronic disabilities that become manifest in adulthood, such as cardiovascular disease, diabetes, and kidney disease [32–35].

Current obstetric practice has relied on the detection and management of growth disorders by estimating fetal weight using 2DUS. Conventional classification of fetal size is based on the pediatric literature from nearly 40 years ago: small (<10th percentile, small for gestational age [SGA]), appropriate (10th–90th percentile, average for gestational age [AGA]), or large (>90th percentile, large for gestational age [LGA]) [36]. Unfortunately, this widely used approach does not distinguish SGA fetuses that are small, but otherwise normal, from other SGA fetuses that are malnourished or have some developmental problem. More sophisticated methods are required for detecting truly malnourished fetuses. If detected early enough, these fetuses may benefit from early intervention for the prevention of pathologic processes that adversely impact health in adult life.

Dudley [37] systematically evaluated 11 different fetal weight estimation models that use common sonographic parameters. No preferred method of fetal weight estimation emerged from this extensive review. This study found that the random error (precision) "remains a major obstacle to confident use in clinical practice, with 95% CI exceeding 14% of birth weight in all studies." Clearly, this review suggests an urgent need to develop more precise fetal weight estimation procedures to guide optimal prenatal care. The most common weight estimation algorithms, however, do not consider fetal soft tissue.

More recently, 3DUS has been reported to improve the accuracy and precision of fetal weight estimation by adding information about soft tissue of the limbs. This approach has been constrained by the amount of time it takes to trace manually the soft tissue borders along the entire fetal limb, especially around the ends of the long bone. Fractional limb volume has been introduced to reduce the time required for an examiner to trace manually the soft tissue borders of the arm or thigh [38].

Technique

A commercially available software tool (4D View, v5.0, GE Healthcare, Milwaukee, Wisconsin) is now capable of measuring fractional limb volume by analyzing a midsection of arm or thigh (Fig. 4A). Fractional limb volume is a subvolume based on 50% of the long bone length. Multiplanar ultrasonographic views (sagittal, coronal, and axial) of the fetal arm or thigh have been obtained using 3DUS. Electronic calipers are manually placed on the ends of the long bone (Fig. 4B). This subvolume is automatically split into five equal disks, each of which is displayed as a corresponding limb section that is manually traced from an axial view (upper right window). After completing the first circular trace around the limb, the cutting plane moves to the second of five total slices that can be measured in a similar manner. The total volume of the five slices equals the fractional limb volume (Fig. 4C). Fractional limb volume measurements take about 2 minutes, are reproducible, and allow the examiner to trace more confidently the soft tissue borders at the center of the limb, where anatomic landmarks are less likely to be obscured by acoustic shadowing.

New fetal weight estimation models that incorporate fractional limb volume throughout pregnancy have now been developed [39]. To date, the most precise fetal weight estimation results have been obtained by using the following function:

$$11.1372\,(BDP^2) - 67.2281\,(BDP) + 1.2175\,(AC^2)$$
$$- 17.3004\,(AC) - 0.0490\,(Tvol^2)$$
$$+ 25.3052\,(TVol) + 285.429$$

where abdominal circumference (*AC*) is, biparietal diameter (*BPD*) is, and fractional thigh volume (*TVol*) is

In a prospective validation study involving 55 fetuses (range: 390 to 5143 g), a greater than twofold improvement was observed in the proportion of infants with a predicted birth weight within 5% of actual birth weight [39]. Fractional arm and thigh volumes have also been applied successfully to individualized fetal growth assessment using the Rossavik fetal growth model [40,41]. Fractional limb volume may provide a directly measured parameter that better reflects the generalized nutritional status of the fetus when compared with estimated fetal weight. Future investigation is required to determine the clinical significance of soft tissue parameters with regards to pregnancy outcome.

The fractional limb volume software should be set at 50% of the diaphyseal bone length, with five slices to define the subvolume. Several considerations should be taken into account for optimal and reproducible fractional limb volume measurements:

1. Volume acquisition of the fetal arm or thigh should be from a sagittal view.

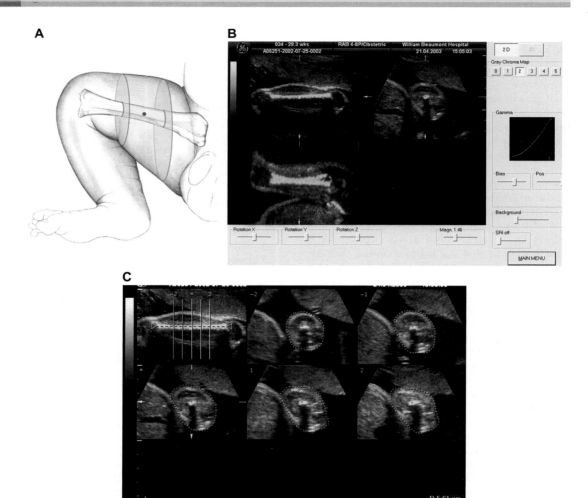

Fig. 4. (*A*) Fractional thigh volume. This soft tissue measurement is based on 50% of the femoral diaphysis length. (*Reproduced from* Lee W, Deter RL, Ebersole JD, et al. Birthweight prediction by 3D ultrsonography: fractional limb volume. J Ultrasound Med 2001;20:1283–92; with permission.) (*B*) Fractional limb volume tool. The original plane of volume acquisition is represented by a magnified view of the femoral diaphysis (*top left window*) A color filter (sepia) has been applied to improve visualization of soft tissue borders. Brightness and contrast are used to optimize image quality. (*C*) Fractional thigh volume. The fractional thigh volume of 25.4 cm³ is calculated by adding the five subvolumes. This measurement can be used with a fetal weight estimation model that also includes abdominal circumference and biparietal diameter.

2. Excessive transducer pressure should be avoided on the maternal abdomen (eg, avoid compression). Fluid around the limb will make it easier for one to visualize soft tissue borders.
3. The limb should be magnified so that it fills a good portion of the screen when preparing for volume acquisition.
4. A sepia color filter can be applied to improve soft tissue contrast.
5. The bias and gain can be used to optimize visualization of soft tissue borders.
6. From the sagittal view, the cutting plane should be dragged back and forth to visualize the quality of soft tissue borders in the axial plane of the limb.

7. The tracing dots should skim the outside of the skin line; some investigators have used a graphics tablet and pen for this procedure.
8. The examiner has the option of exporting the image panel as a JPEG file. This image can be examined for quality control, be made into a slide, or sent to a colleague for a second opinion.

Tissue perfusion

Three-dimensional power Doppler angiography (3D-PDA) combines 3DUS and VOCAL to estimate organ tissue perfusion. Pairleitner and coworkers [42] introduced this technique for quantifying

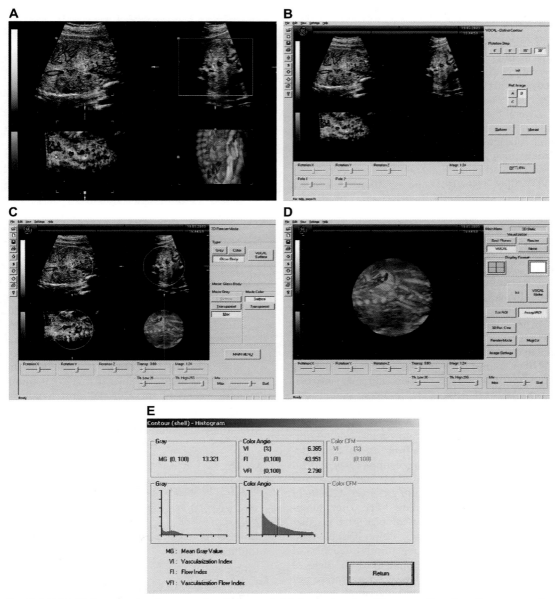

Fig. 5. (*A*) Multiplanar and volume-rendered views of fetal vessels using 3D power Doppler ultrasonography. (*B*)Placement of green triangular markers along body wall (*top left*) to define center of rotation for VOCAL technique. (*C*) Segmentation of circular volume contains both colored and gray-scale voxels (*lower right image*). (*D*) Segmentation of circular volume contains both colored and gray-scale voxels. (*E*) Histogram analysis for vascular flow indices.

low-velocity blood flow in adnexal masses. Studies have carefully examined the reproducibility of 3D vascular flow indices because many factors could potentially affect these measurements (eg, system gain, transducer frequency, pulse repetition frequency, and acoustic power). For example, Raine-Fenning and colleagues [43] acquired 20 ovarian and 20 endometrial volumes from 40 different patients at various stages of in vitro fertilization treatment. The intraobserver reliability was extremely high and reliability was no different between observers for vascular indices within the ovary or endometrium. The interobserver reliability of these ovarian, endometrial, and subendometrial measurements was very good, with a mean intra-class correlation coefficient of above 0.985. In another investigation, they confirmed that these techniques can be used reliably among examiners for uterine vascularity studies [44]. Another study examined 40 women with 3D-PDA to evaluate the interobserver reproducibility of vascular indices in this manner [45]. Endometrial and subendometrial vascularity indices were associated with a mean intraclass correlation coefficient that was greater than 0.84.

Several investigators have used these 3D vascular flow indices for several gynecologic conditions. Pan and colleagues [46] examined differences in ovarian stromal flow in patients who had polycystic ovarian syndrome. The vascularization flow index (VFI), flow index (FI), and vascularization index (VI), were significantly higher ($P<.05$) in affected women, compared with women having normal ovaries. They subsequently documented lower Doppler indices of ovarian stromal blood flow in women who were poor responders to gonadotropins during in vitro fertilization therapy [47]. Raine-Fenning and coworkers [48] examined periodic changes in endometrial development and subendometrial vascularity during the normal menstrual cycle and found significantly reduced 3D vascular flow indices in women with unexplained subfertility.

Other studies have applied 3D vascular flow indices for the fetal liver, brain, kidneys, and placenta [49–52]. All flow indices significantly increased over time with advancing pregnancy. Merce and colleagues [53] evaluated the reproducibility of placental vascular flow indices on 30 normal singleton pregnancies from 14 to 40 weeks, menstrual age. All 3D power Doppler vascular indices (VI, FI, and VFI) showed a correlation greater than 0.85, with a better intraobserver agreement for the flow indices (FI and VFI). They subsequently described increases of placental vascular flow indices over time [54]. Power Doppler settings included a pulsed repetition frequency of 600 Hz; wall filter 40 Hz; and fixed 35° field of view, although the overall gain settings were not reported. The FI, reflecting placental flow, increased in a linear and progressive manner, as compared with VI (number of placental vessels) that increased up to the 30th week. The VI maintained a plateau up to the 37th week and decreased afterwards.

Technique

The following steps demonstrate a typical approach for acquiring volume data sets by 3D-PDA and for analyzing a volume of interest by VOCAL using histograms for flow vascularization indices:

Step 1. Obtain a volume acquisition by 3D power Doppler ultrasonography, using standardized presets. A multiplanar view of the fetal abdomen is displayed (Fig. 5A). Vascular structures and vertical spine are seen in the lower right window.

Step 2. Place the two contour points on the main rotation axis (Fig. 5B) to define a volume of interest (upper left window).

Step 3. The outline of the volume of interest can be isolated by either an automated spherical or a manual contouring procedure. For demonstration purposes, a spherical subvolume is created around the two initial contour points used to define the initial volume boundaries. The "glass body" rendering mode displays a spherical subvolume (Fig. 5C).

Step 4. This spherical subvolume (enlarged) consists of a proportionate number of quantifiable gray-scale voxels and colored voxels that correspond to blood flow (Fig. 5D).

Step 5. The VIEW pull-down menu is selected for HISTOGRAM to compute the gray-scale or power Doppler distribution within the defined subvolume. The gray-scale and Doppler-based values are normalized to maximal incidence from a scale of 0 to 100 on the vertical axis. The horizontal axis represents the gray-scale intensity values (0 to 255) or amplitude values of the Doppler shift frequency (Fig. 5E).

The following parameters are described in Box 1.

Box 1:   3D power Doppler vascular indices

VI = Vascularization Index (standardized range 0 to 100)
Number of color voxels in relation to total number of voxels

Example:

    Number of color voxels = 1000
    Total number of voxels = 5000
    VI = 1000/5000 = 0.2%

FI = Flow Index (standardized range 0 to 100)
Average intensity value of color voxels contained in the volume.

Example:

    500 color voxels have a very high intensity = 80
    500 color voxels have a lower intensity = 20
    [(500 * 80) + (500*20)]/1000 total voxels = FI = 50
    or 0.5%

VFI = Vascularization Flow Index
VFI = (VI *FI)/100

Example:

    VFI = .2 × .5 = .10 or 10%

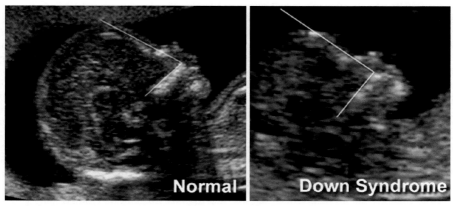

Fig. 6. Frontal maxillary facial angle in a chromosomally normal fetus (*left*) and one with trisomy 21 (*right*). (*Courtesy of* Dr. Jiri Sonek, Dayton, OH.)

Detection of Down syndrome

The well-known midfacial hypoplasia that occurs with Down syndrome appears to be present in affected fetuses as early as 11 0/7 to 13 6/7 weeks, menstrual age [55]. Sonek and colleagues [56] have recently examined the usefulness of a new facial angle measurement, the frontomaxillary facial (FMF) angle, for detecting fetuses at risk for trisomy 21 (**Fig. 6**) [54]. In this study, 3DUS was used to acquire volumes of the fetal head in 100 fetuses with trisomy 21 and 300 normal fetuses at 11 to 13^{+6} weeks. Fetuses with Down syndrome had a significantly greater FMF angle than normal fetuses (mean 88.7°, range 75.4°–104° versus mean 78.1°, range 66.6°–89.5°, P<.001). Sixty-nine percent of the trisomy 21 fetuses had an FMF angle greater than the 95th percentile (85°) of the euploid population. Forty percent of the trisomy 21 fetuses had an FMF angle above the upper limit of the range of angles (90°) of the euploid population. The measurement of FMF angles, as an index of midfacial hypoplasia, may be an important adjunctive technique for prenatal screening for trisomy 21.

Summary

This article summarizes some of the quantitative applications offered by 3DUS. Volume sonography provides much more than surface and volume-rendered reconstructions of fetal anatomy. Quantitative analysis is now possible by allowing the standardization of distance, angle, area, and volume measurements. Optimal uses of these analytic approaches are emerging as software tools become more sophisticated and as we begin to apply these new capabilities to various clinical problems. Health care providers should be aware of these emerging capabilities and their potential applications.

References

[1] Benacerraf BR, Benson CB, Abuhamad AZ, et al. Three- and 4-dimensional ultrasound in obstetrics and gynecology: proceedings of the American Institute of Ultrasound in Medicine Consensus Conference. J Ultrasound Med 2005; 24:1587–97.

[2] Gonçalves LF, Lee W, Espinoza J, et al. Three- and 4-dimensional ultrasound in obstetric practice: does it help? J Ultrasound Med 2005;24: 1599–624.

[3] Billingsley FC. Digital video processing at JPL. In: Turner EB, editor, Electronic imaging techniques, SPIE proceedings, vol. 3. Bellingham (WA): Society for Photocoptical Instrumentation Engineers; 1964. p. 15.

[4] Billingsley FC. Processing ranger and mariner photography (capabilities of lunar televison image converter system used for digital processing of ranger and mariner pictures). SPIE Journal 1966;4:147–55.

[5] Kollias SS, Goldstein RB, Cogen PH, et al. Prenatally detected myelomeningoceles: sonographic accuracy in estimation of the spinal level. Radiology 1992;185:109–12.

[6] Bruner JP, Tulipan N, Dabrowiak ME, et al. Upper level of the spina bifida defect: how good are we? Ultrasound Obstet Gynecol 2004;24:612–7.

[7] Mueller GM, Weiner CP, Yankowitz J. Three-dimensional ultrasound in the evaluation of fetal head and spine anomalies. Obstet Gynecol 1996;88:372–8.

[8] Riccabona M, Johnson D, Pretorius DH, et al. Three dimensional ultrasound: display modalities in the fetal spine and thorax. Eur J Radiol 1996;22:141–5.

[9] Johnson DD, Pretorius DH, Riccabona M, et al. Three-dimensional ultrasound of the fetal spine. Obstet Gynecol 1997;89:434–8.

[10] Leung KY, Ngai CSW, Chan BC, et al. Three-dimensional extended imaging: a new display modality for three-dimensional ultrasound

examination. Ultrasound Obstet Gynecol 2005; 26:244–51.

[11] Lee W, Chaiworapongsa T, Romero R, et al. A diagnostic approach for the evaluation of spina bifida by three-dimensional ultrasonography. J Ultrasound Med 2002;21:619–26.

[12] Online Mendelian Inheritance in Man (OMIM database). Available at: http://www.ncbi.nlm.nih.gov/entrez/query.fcgi?db=OMIM. Accessed October 14, 2006.

[13] Vettraino IM, Lee W, Bronsteen RA, et al. Clinical outcome of fetuses with sonographic diagnosis of isolated micrognathia. Obstet Gynecol 2003; 102:801–5.

[14] Lee W, McNie B, Chaiworapongsa T, et al. Three-dimensional ultrasonographic presentation of micrognathia. J Ultrasound Med 2002;21: 775–81.

[15] Wulfsberg EA, Leana-Cox J, Neri G. Reply to "What's in a name? The 22q11.2 deletion". [Letter to the editor]. Am J Med Genet 1997;72: 248–9.

[16] Arvystas M, Shprintzen RJ. Craniofacial morphology in the velocardio-facial syndrome. J Craniofac Genet Dev Biol 1984;4:39–45.

[17] Rotten D, Levaillant JM, Martinez H, et al. The fetal mandible: a 2D and 3D sonographic approach to the diagnosis of retrognathia and micrognathia. Ultrasound Obstet Gynecol 2002; 19:122–30.

[18] Riccabona M, Nelson TR, Pretorius DH. Three-dimensional ultrasound: accuracy of distance and volume measurements. Ultrasound Obstet Gynecol 1996;7:429–34.

[19] Bordes A, Bory AM, Benchaib M, et al. Reproducibility of transvaginal three-dimensional endometrial volume measurements with virtual organ computer-aided analysis (VOCAL) during ovarian stimulation. Ultrasound Obstet Gynecol 2002;9:76–80.

[20] Raine-Fenning NJ, Campbell B, Collier J, et al. The reproducibility of endometrial volume acquisition and measurement with the VOCAL-imaging program. Ultrasound Obstet Gynecol 2002;19:69–75.

[21] Raine-Fenning NJ, Clewes JS, Kendall NR, et al. The interobserver reliability and validity of volume calculation from three-dimensional ultrasound datasets in the in vitro setting. Ultrasound Obstet Gynecol 2003;21:283–91.

[22] Lee W, Deter RL, McNie B, et al. Quantitative and morphological assessment of early gestational sacs using three-dimensional ultrasonography. Ultrasound Obstet Gynecol 2006;28:255–60.

[23] Bhat AH, Corbett VN, Liu R, et al. Validation of volume and mass assessments for human fetal heart imaging by 4-dimensional spatiotemporal image correlation echocardiography: in vitro balloon model experiments. J Ultrasound Med 2004;23:1151–9.

[24] Peralta CF, Cavoretto P, Csapo B, et al. Lung and heart volumes by three-dimensional ultrasound in normal fetuses at 12-32 weeks' gestation. Ultrasound Obstet Gynecol 2006;27:128–33.

[25] Hafner E, Metzenbauer M, Dillinger-Paller B, et al. Correlation of first trimester placental volume and second trimester uterine artery Doppler flow. Placenta 2001;22:729–34.

[26] Falcon O, Peralta CF, Cavoretto P, et al. Fetal trunk and head volume in chromosomally abnormal fetuses at 11+0 to 13+6 weeks of gestation. Ultrasound Obstet Gynecol 2005;26:517–20.

[27] Falcon O, Wegrzyn P, Faro C, et al. Gestational sac volume measured by three-dimensional ultrasound at 11 to 13+6 weeks of gestation: relation to chromosomal defects. Ultrasound Obstet Gynecol 2005;25:546–50.

[28] Gadelha PS, Da Costa AG, Filho FM, et al. Amniotic fluid volumetry by three-dimensional ultrasonography during the first trimester of pregnancy. Ultrasound Med Biol 2006;32: 1135–9.

[29] Kalache KD, Espinoza J, Chaiworapongsa T, et al. Three-dimensional ultrasound fetal lung volume measurement: a systematic study comparing the multiplanar method with the rotational (VOCAL) technique. Ultrasound Obstet Gynecol 2003;21:111–8.

[30] Ruano R, Martinovic J, Dommergues M, et al. Accuracy of fetal lung volume assessed by three-dimensional sonography. Ultrasound Obstet Gynecol 2005;26:725–30.

[31] Ruano R, Joubin L, Aubry MC, et al. A nomogram of fetal lung volumes estimated by 3-dimensional ultrasonography using the rotational technique (virtual organ computer-aided analysis). J Ultrasound Med 2006;25:701–9.

[32] Barker D. The midwife, the coincidence, and the hypothesis. BMJ 2003;327:1428–30.

[33] Reyes L, Manalich R. Long-term consequences of low birth weight. Kidney Int Suppl 2005;97: S107–11.

[34] McMillen IC, Robinson JS. Developmental origins of the metabolic syndrome: prediction, plasticity, and programming. Physiol Rev 2005; 85:571–633.

[35] Plagemann A. Perinatal nutrition and hormone-dependent programming of food intake. Horm Res 2006;65:83–9.

[36] Battaglia FC, Lubchenco LO. A practical application of newborn infants by weight and gestational age. J Pediatr 1967;71:159–63.

[37] Dudley NJ. A systematic review of the ultrasound estimation of fetal weight. Ultrasound Obstet Gynecol 2005;25:80–9.

[38] Lee W, Deter RL, Ebersole JD, et al. Birthweight prediction by 3D ultrasonography: fractional limb volume. J Ultrasound Med 2001;20:1283–92.

[39] Lee W, Balasubramaniam M, Deter RL, et al. Soft tissue parameters improve the precision of fetal weight estimation [abstract]. Ultrasound Obstet Gynecol 2006;28:389.

[40] Lee W, Deter RL, McNie B, et al. Individualized growth assessment of fetal soft tissue using

fractional thigh volume. Ultrasound Obstet Gynecol 2004;24:766–74.

[41] Lee W, Deter RL, McNie B, et al. The fetal arm: individualized growth assessment in normal pregnancies. J Ultrasound Med 2005;24:817–28.

[42] Pairleitner H, Steiner H, Hasenoehrl G, et al. Three-dimensional power Doppler sonography: imaging and quantifying blood flow and vascularization. Ultrasound Obstet Gynecol 1999;17:201–6.

[43] Raine-Fenning NJ, Campbell BK, Clewes JS, et al. The reliability of virtual organ computer-aided analysis (VOCAL) for the semi quantification of ovarian, endometrial and subendometrial perfusion. Ultrasound Obstet Gynecol 2003;22:633–9.

[44] Raine-Fenning NJ, Campbell BK, Clewes JS, et al. The interobserver reliability of three-dimensional power Doppler data acquisition within the female pelvis. Ultrasound Obstet Gynecol 2004;23:501–8.

[45] Alcazar JL, Merce LT, Manero MG, et al. Endometrial volume and vascularity measurements by transvaginal 3-dimensional ultrasonography and power Doppler angiography in stimulated and tumoral endometria: an interobserver reproducibility study. J Ultrasound Med 2005;24:1091–8.

[46] Pan HA, Wu MH, Cheng YC, et al. Quantification of Doppler signal in polycystic ovary syndrome using three-dimensional power Doppler ultrasonography: a possible new marker for diagnosis. Hum Reprod 2002;17:201–6.

[47] Pan HA, Wu MH, Cheng YC, et al. Quantification of ovarian stromal Doppler signals in poor responders undergoing in vitro fertilization with three-dimensional power Doppler ultrasonography. Am J Obstet Gynecol 2004;190:338–44.

[48] Raine-Fenning NJ, Campbell BK, Kendall NR, et al. Endometrial and subendometrial perfusion are impaired in women with unexplained subfertility. Hum Reprod 2004;19:2605–14.

[49] Chang CH, Yu CH, Ko HC, et al. Assessment of normal fetal liver blood flow using quantitative three-dimensional power Doppler ultrasound. Ultrasound Med Biol 2003;29:943–9.

[50] Chang CH, Yu CH, Ko HC, et al. Three-dimensional power Doppler ultrasound for the assessment of the fetal brain blood flow in normal gestation. Ultrasound Med Biol 2003;29:1273–9.

[51] Chang CH, Yu CH, Ko HC, et al. Quantitative three-dimensional power Doppler sonography for assessment of the fetal renal blood flow in normal gestation. Ultrasound Med Biol 2003;29:929–33.

[52] Yu CH, Chang CH, Ko HC, et al. Assessment of placental fractional moving blood volume using quantitative three-dimensional power doppler ultrasound. Ultrasound Med Biol 2003;29:19–23.

[53] Merce LT, Barco MJ, Bau S. Reproducibility of the study of placental vascularization by three-dimensional power Doppler. J Perinat Med 2004;32:228–33.

[54] Merce LT, Barco MJ, Bau S, et al. Assessment of placental vascularization by three-dimensional power Doppler "vascular biopsy" in normal pregnancies. Croat Med J 2005;46:765–71.

[55] Dagklis T, Borenstein M, Peralta CF, et al. Three-dimensional evaluation of mid-facial hypoplasia in fetuses with trisomy 21 at 11 + 0 to 13 + 6 weeks of gestation. Ultrasound Obstet Gynecol 2006;28:261–5.

[56] Sonek J, Borenstein M, Dagklis T, et al. Fronto maxillary facial angle in fetuses with trisomy 21 at 11 − 13 + 6 weeks. Am J Obstet Gynecol 2007;196(271):e1–4.

ELSEVIER
SAUNDERS

ULTRASOUND CLINICS

Ultrasound Clin 2 (2007) 217–244

Ultrasound of the Fetal Brain

Ana Monteagudo, MD*, Ilan E. Timor-Tritsch, MD

Ultrasound examination of the fetal central nervous system (CNS) distinguishes itself from the sonographic evaluation of all other organs or organ systems, such as the limbs, kidneys, heart, and liver, to name just a few, in that the aforementioned structures are in place, almost in their final developmental form, from the latter part of the first trimester, with minute or no substantial changes as the pregnancy progresses. During the course of the pregnancy, all that is happening with these organs or organ systems is that they undergo changes in their size (ie, they grow). In contrast, the CNS (mainly the fetal brain) undergoes significant changes, not only in size but in the shape of its different anatomic regions. These changes of size and shape follow a well-defined timeline and can be recognized sonographically. The developmental milestones of the CNS from the time of its first sonographic detection (by 8 postmenstrual weeks) to term can, and should, be taken into consideration when a fetal neurosonogram is performed. To evaluate the fetal brain accurately, it is imperative to know the exact postmenstrual age of the fetus. A 2- to 4-week error in dating because of uncertain last menstrual period or conception date may make the difference between diagnosing a normal brain structure or its anomalous development.

This article is not meant to be an all-inclusive encyclopedia of brain anomalies. Its main purpose is to describe a systematic approach to the evaluation of the fetal brain. The systematic approach is illustrated by discussing at length the differential diagnosis of two important sonographic findings, namely ventriculomegaly and an enlarged posterior fossa, and by touching on other important brain abnormalities.

Sono-embryology of the fetal brain

The following paragraph is not meant to be a detailed description of the developmental changes that occur in the fetal brain during gestation. Its scope is to give the reader a quick reference as to the gestational age when major brain structures can be seen by transabdominal or transvaginal sonography.

The embryonic head can be imaged as a separate entity from the embryonic pole late in the seventh postmenstrual week of gestation. Within the head, a single round anechoic cavity (rhombencephalon) almost completely fills the embryonic head. At 8 postmenstrual weeks, sagittal, axial, and coronal sections of the embryonic brain can be obtained. On the sagittal view, the embryonic head reveals four sequential, interconnecting anechoic structures. From anterior to posterior, these anechoic structures correspond to the telencephalon (future lateral ventricles), diencephalon (future third ventricle),

Department of Obstetrics and Gynecology, NYU School of Medicine, 530 First Avenue, NB9N26, New York, NY 10016, USA
* Corresponding author.
E-mail address: ana.monteagudo@med.nyu.edu (A. Monteagudo).

1556-858X/07/$ – see front matter © 2007 Elsevier Inc. All rights reserved.
ultrasound.theclinics.com

doi:10.1016/j.cult.2007.07.003

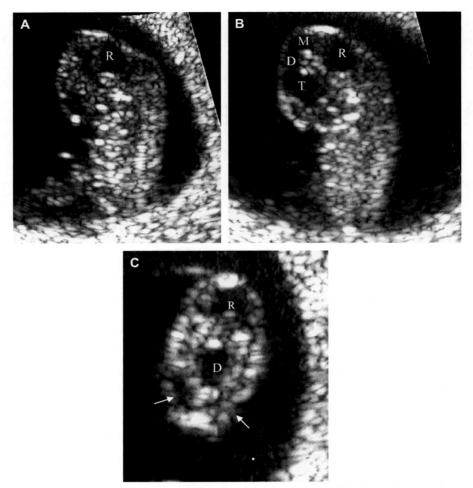

Fig. 1. The developing fetal brain at 8 postmenstrual weeks. (*A, B*) Sagittal sections, showing the sites of the future brain structures. (*C*) An axial section. The arrows point to the telencephalic vesicle. (D, diencephalon; M, myelencephalon; R, rhombencephalon; T, telencephalon.)

mesencephalon (future aqueduct), and metencephalon (future fourth ventricle), respectively. If a posterior coronal section is obtained, the rhombencephalon is seen as a single round anechoic structure filling almost the entire head (Fig. 1).

The ninth postmenstrual week brings several important developments. The falx cerebri and the choroid plexus become sonographically apparent (Fig. 2). A right and a left hemisphere are now apparent. At this time in pregnancy, the appearance of the choroid plexuses within the ventricle has been likened to a butterfly with its wings spread open (Figs. 3 and 4).

During the 10th to 13th postmenstrual week, the third ventricle can be seen as an anechoic midline structure between the echogenic wings of the choroid plexus. On sagittal and axial sections of the

brain, the anterior horn of the lateral ventricle appears prominent (see Fig. 4), and within the posterior fossa, the cerebellum, as such, appears for the first time.

After the 14th postmenstrual week, the cerebral cortex becomes "thicker" and can be imaged clearly. The cerebellar hemispheres and the upper part of the cerebellar vermis, which is located between the two cerebellar hemispheres, are evident (Fig. 5). Starting around 16 postmenstrual weeks, on an axial transthalamic section, the cavum septi pellucidi can be consistently imaged below the falx cerebri and superior to the thalami (Fig. 6).

After 18 postmenstrual weeks, the corpus callosum almost completes its development and can be seen, using the median section. However, only after the 20th postmenstrual week can the normally and

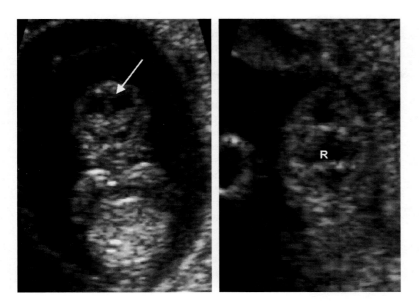

Fig. 2. Coronal and semi-axial planes of a fetal brain at 9 postmenstrual weeks. The arrow points to the falx cerebri. (R, rhombencephalon.)

fully developed corpus callosum and pericallosal artery be seen consistently (Fig. 7). Similarly, because at this age the cerebellum is fully developed, the entire cerebellar vermis should be seen (Fig. 8). Parasagittal sections reveal each lateral ventricle, choroid plexus, and lateral (sylvian) fissure (Fig. 9). Using transabdominal sonography, the posterior fossa can be imaged best by placing the transducer over the suture, between the occipital and parietal bone (see Fig. 8C).

Most of the fetal gyri and sulci develop later in gestation and can be seen sonographically on the medial surface of the hemispheres. The first cortical surface structures seen at 18 to 20 postmenstrual weeks are the cingulate sulcus and parieto-occipital fissure (calcar avis). However, the insula can be seen as a lateral indentation on axial sections of the fetal brain from about 18 postmenstrual weeks (Fig. 10) [1,2].

The basic examination of the fetal brain

The basic examination [3] can be performed by transabdominal sonography, using three axial sections of the head during the late first, second, or third trimester of the pregnancy. This examination includes imaging several brain structures and obtaining important biometric measurements. The brain structures sought are lateral ventricles, cavum septi pellucidi, thalami, cerebellum, cisterna magna, and spine. The biometric measurements performed after examining the head shape are the biparietal diameter, head circumference, and occipitofrontal diameter; the atrium of the lateral ventricle at the level of the choroid plexus, the transcerebellar diameter, and the depth of the cisterna magna are also measured.

In the transventricular axial plane, the landmarks from anterior-to-posterior are as follows: the cavum septi pellucidi, flanked on each side by the anterior horn of the lateral ventricle; and posteriorly, the posterior horn of the lateral ventricle, which contains the hyperechoic choroid plexus (see Fig. 10A). The walls of the ventricles are echogenic and are demarcated clearly by the fluid contained within the ventricle. At this level, the lateral ventricles are measured at the widest part, at the level of the glomus of the choroid plexus. The calipers are placed perpendicular to the ventricle in the inner

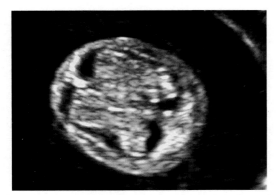

Fig. 3. At 9.5 postmenstrual weeks, the choroid plexuses assure the shape of a butterfly.

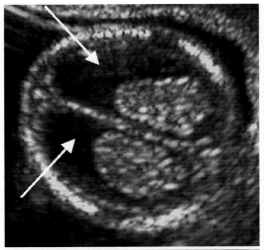

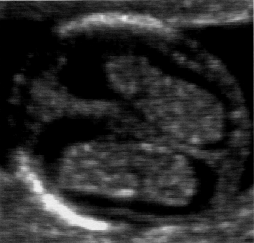

Fig. 4. Note that at 9 to 13 postmenstrual weeks, the choroid plexuses do not fill the lateral ventricles, which is normal at this gestational age. Arrows point to the anterior horns of the lateral ventricle.

aspect of the wall of the lateral ventricle. A measurement of up to 10 mm is deemed normal.

Inferior to this plane is the transthalamic plane. The landmarks from anterior-to-posterior are the frontal horns of the lateral ventricle, the cavum septi pellucidi, the thalami, and the hippocampal gyri (see Fig. 10B). It is at this level that most of the biometric measurements of the head are obtained, namely, the biparietal diameter, head circumference, and occipitofrontal diameter.

The transcerebellar axial plane is inferior to the transthalamic plane and is tilted posteriorly to image the posterior fossa adequately. The landmarks from anterior-to-posterior in this plane are the frontal horns of the lateral ventricles, the cavum septi pellucidi, the thalami, the cerebellum, and the

cisterna magna (see Fig. 10C). A cisterna magna measuring greater than 10 mm is considered abnormal; also considered abnormal is lack of visualization of the cisterna magna.

If any of the structures included in the basic examination cannot be visualized, or if the biometric measurements obtained are outside the realm of normalcy, a targeted scan of the fetal brain or a detailed fetal neurosonogram needs to be performed. This scan assesses the brain in greater detail. It can be performed transabdominally; however, because the aim of the detailed neurosonogram is to visualize the relevant brain structures in all three scanning planes, additional ultrasound techniques should be used. The transvaginal scanning approach enables the coronal and sagittal sections to be visualized, provided the fetus is in cephalic presentation. In addition, the transabdominal and transvaginal approaches can be enhanced significantly by using three-dimensional (3D) or volume sonography.

The targeted fetal neurosonogram

During the basic examination of the brain, the pertinent brain sections in the axial plane are seen and described (Fig. 11A). During the more extended, detailed fetal neurosonogram [3], the emphasis is on the addition of coronal and sagittal planes. The easiest way to obtain these planes, if the fetus is in cephalic presentation, is by way of the transvaginal route. If the fetus is in breech presentation, an attempt can be made to obtain the above sections transabdominally, with the higher-frequency transvaginal probe placed into the maternal umbilicus, which will result in images with high resolution. If this procedure does not yield diagnostic quality images, an external cephalic version can be attempted. When scanning transvaginally, the sections are obtained through the anterior fontanelle (Fig. 11B) or one of the sutures of the skull (see Fig. 8C); therefore, both hemispheres are assessed adequately and can be compared with each other. Although many coronal and sagittal sections are possible, concentrating on four coronal and two sagittal sections yields valuable additional information, in addition to that obtained by the axial sections [1,4]. In most cases, these sections are sufficient to arrive at a diagnosis.

The coronal planes are shown in Fig. 12. The most important coronal planes from anterior-to-posterior are the transfrontal plane, transcaudate plane, transthalamic plane, and transcerebellar plane (see Fig. 12) [4]. The landmarks for the transfrontal plane are the interhemispheric fissure, which equally divides the right and left hemispheres, and the anterior horns of the lateral ventricles; the bony structures seen are the sphenoidal

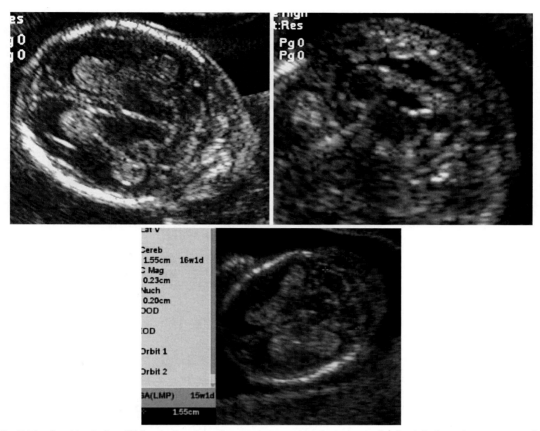

Fig. 5. The fetal brain is sufficiently developed at 15 postmenstrual weeks. A tilted axial plane demonstrates the choroid plexuses and the forming posterior fossa.

bone and orbits. In the transcaudate plane, the structures seen from superior to inferior are the interhemispheric fissure, the hypoechoic horizontal lines of the corpus callosum, the anechoic triangular-shaped cavum septi pellucidi (flanked on both

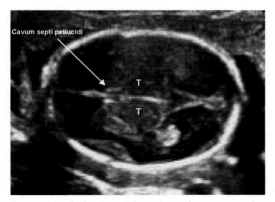

Fig. 6. Transthalamic axial section. The arrow points to the cavum septi pellucidi. The two thalami are also imaged on this plane. (T, thalmai.)

sides by the anechoic frontal horns of the lateral ventricles), and the caudate nucleus. Bilaterally, close to the bones of the cranium, the indentations of the insula are apparent. Moving posteriorly, the next plane is the transthalamic plane. This view is an important one because many pathologies can be identified by studying this plane carefully. The structures, from superior to inferior, are similar to those viewed in the previous section but, instead of the caudate nucleus, the thalami are seen. The third ventricle, situated between the thalami on either side, is seldom seen in a normal brain. If prominent, it is usually part of a generally dilated ventricular system. The transcerebellar plane is the most posterior plane. The structures seen superior to inferior are the interhemispheric fissure and the occipital horns of the lateral ventricles, which on this plane are devoid of choroid plexus and appear round, rendering this plane the owl's face configuration. Inferior, below the tentorium, the contents of the posterior fossa are seen (the cerebellum, the vermis, and the cisterna magna).

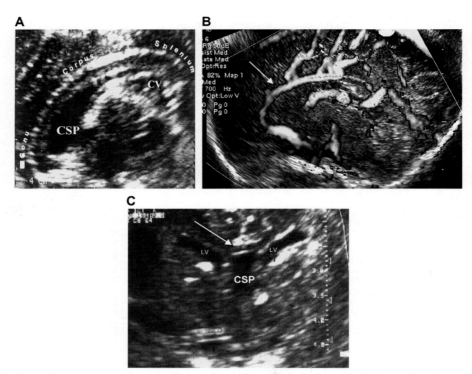

Fig. 7. At 19 to 20 postmenstrual weeks, the corpus callosum is fully formed. (*A*) A median plane shows the C-shaped corpus callosum and the cavum septi pellucid (CSP) below it. (*B*) The pericallosal artery follows the corpus callosum from above. (*C*) On a coronal section, the lateral ventricles (LV), the CSP, and the corpus callosum (*arrow*) are seen.

The sagittal planes (Fig. 13) are the median plane and the two left and right parasagittal planes. The median plane is one of the most important and diagnostically useful planes because it depicts the important midline structures of

> Corpus callosum. The normal corpus callosum is hypoechoic and its shape is similar to a "C" that is lying horizontally, with the curved part superior. The corpus callosum has several parts to it from anterior to posterior: the rostrum (beak), the genu (knee), the corpus (body of the corpus callosum), and the splenium (tail).
> Pericallosal artery (using Doppler evaluation, located superior to the corpus callosum)
> Third ventricle
> Tela choroidea covering the thalamus (locus of the germinal matrix prone to hemorrhage)
> Quadrigeminal plate and cistern (frequent location of arachnoid cysts)
> Vermis of the cerebellum
> Fourth ventricle
> Cisterna magna

The right and left parasagittal planes reveal the anterior, posterior, and, at times, inferior horns of the lateral ventricle (seen as an inverted "C") containing the echogenic choroid plexus.

Three-dimensional fetal neurosonography

Three-dimensional sonography or volume sonography can simplify the process of obtaining the serial sagittal and coronal sections [5,6]. The main difference between the sections or planes obtained by two-dimensional (2D) transvaginal sonography and 3D transvaginal sonography is that when using 2D sonography, all the sections arise from a single point, usually the anterior fontanelle fanning out in a radial fashion, and are oblique to one another. In contrast, when using 3D transvaginal sonography, the sections obtained from the saved volume are parallel to each other, similar to those obtained by CT or MR imaging. Another difference between 2D and 3D sonography is that with 3D sonography, a reconstructed axial plane is possible; therefore, all three scanning planes can be imaged on the screen

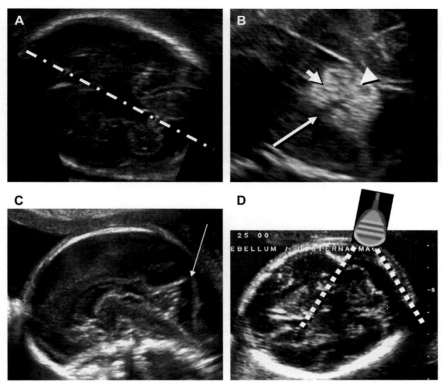

Fig. 8. After 18 postmenstrual weeks, the cerebellum is fully formed. (*A*) Tilted axial section. (*B*) Median section. The vermian lobes are separated by fissures (*arrowhead and short arrow*). The fourth ventricle is marked by a long arrow. (*C*) Median section depicts a wide view with the normal vermian structure. The normally positioned tentorium and torcular are marked with a white arrow. (*D*) Placing an abdominal transducer over the suture between the occipita and parietal bones enables a clear view of the posterior fossa.

simultaneously. While scanning the fetal brain using 3D sonography, a volume of the fetal head can be obtained transvaginally through the fontanelle or the sagittal suture (see Fig. 11B) if the fetus is in cephalic presentation. Once the volume is saved, the following display modalities can be used to obtain additional information:

Multiplanar imaging (orthogonal planes): displays the three scanning planes (sagittal,

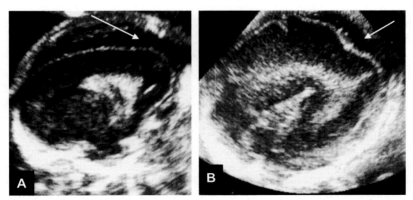

Fig. 9. (*A*) Parasagittal section shows the anterior and posterior horns and the choroid plexus. (*B*) Extremely lateral parasagittal section across the insula. The arrows for both figures point to the anterior fontanelle.

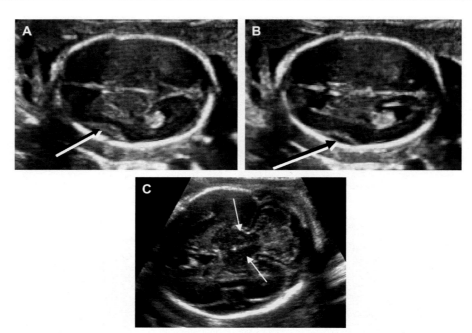

Fig. 10. The insula (*black arrows*) starts to fold in at around 18 weeks and can be seen on the axial planes of the two subsequent sections (*A* and *B*). (*C*) A slightly "lower" axial section showing the superior pedunculi (*white arrows*).

coronal, and axial) that are simultaneously displayed at right angles to each other on the monitor. The user can scroll to navigate in a continuous fashion through each plane. If the volume is obtained either in a coronal or a sagittal plane, the axial plane generated is a reconstructed plane (Fig. 14).

Tomographic display: allows visualization of multiple parallel slices at different spacing through a volume. All subsequent sections can be display at the same time on the screen; therefore, serial sections of any of the planes are similar to those seen by CT or MR imaging (Fig. 15).

3D sono-angiography: enables selective imaging of blood vessels after a 3D acquisition of a power or Color Doppler-containing volume (Fig. 16).

"Thick-slice" display: selected area of the volume is collapsed into a 2D image (Fig. 17) for an enhanced edge or contrast detection.

Radiograph, maximum ("bone") or transparency mode: allows selective imaging of the fetal skeleton (Fig. 18). Therefore, anomalies of the bony skeleton are highlighted. Its use in scanning the fetal head is that of defining the bony skull and its sutures.

Inversion mode: selected fluid-filled areas of the acquired volume can be "inverted";

therefore, the areas that were initially anechoic become echogenic. The on-screen appearance is that of a cast representing the fluid-filled space, in this case the lateral ventricles (Fig. 19).

Surface rendering: widely recognized, even by lay people. The surface features can be seen and recognized as resembling a photograph (eg, the face), which is useful because in several situations, brain anomalies are associated with facial dysmorphism, such as in alobar holoprosencephaly.

Brain anomalies

Ventriculomegaly

One of the more common problems detected during the basic examination is the lateral ventricles measuring more than the upper limits of normal, namely more than 10 mm. How do we work up this sonographic finding?

1. Complete the basic examination of the head using transabdominal sonography. Perform a detailed anatomic survey of the fetus, with special emphasis on the fetal spine. Determine the fetal gender.

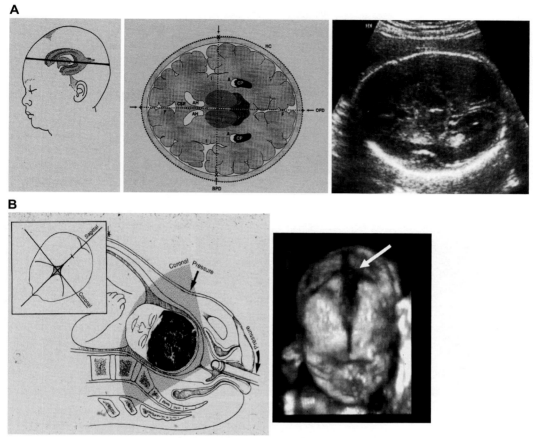

Fig. 11. Transabdominal and transvaginal scanning routes. (*A*) The plane of the biparietal diameter. The ultrasound picture is generated using this plane. It depicts the lateral ventricles, the pedunculi and the walls of the cavum septi pellucid, usually seen using transabdominal ultrasound. (*B*) The technique of transvaginal fetal neuroscan. The widely open fontanelles (*arrow*) and sutures shown in the 3D image are used as "windows" to image the fetal brain.

2. Obtain a short history and, if possible, the results of the first or second trimester maternal serum screen for aneuploidy or fetal karyotype.
3. Perform the detailed and targeted fetal neurosonogram, with special emphasis on the median section of the brain.

Ventriculomegaly is a generic, all-inclusive term for dilatation of the lateral ventricles. If the cerebrospinal fluid is under pressure, the appropriate term is hydrocephaly. The term "ventriculomegaly" is not meant to indicate a diagnosis. It is, rather, a sign of an underlying pathology. It is usually the presenting sign or common final pathway of many chromosomal or nonchromosomal brain anomalies.

In this article, the authors do not include a detailed description of ventriculomegaly's causes and clinical implications. The images presented,

obtained by different sonographic techniques, should constitute examples of their features (Fig. 20).

Dilation of the lateral ventricles can be a clue to several pathologies, such as spina bifida and agenesis of the corpus callosum (ACC). The authors discuss the pathologies that must be excluded when evaluating a fetus with dilation of the lateral ventricles.

Spinal dysraphism (spina bifida)
In spina bifida (see Fig. 20), the basic examination, in addition to demonstrating the spinal pathology and dilatation of the lateral ventricles, may reveal the abnormal head shape (Fig. 21) (the "lemon sign"); the abnormally shaped cerebellum (the "banana sign"); and the obliterated cisterna magna, which cannot be measured because the cerebellum

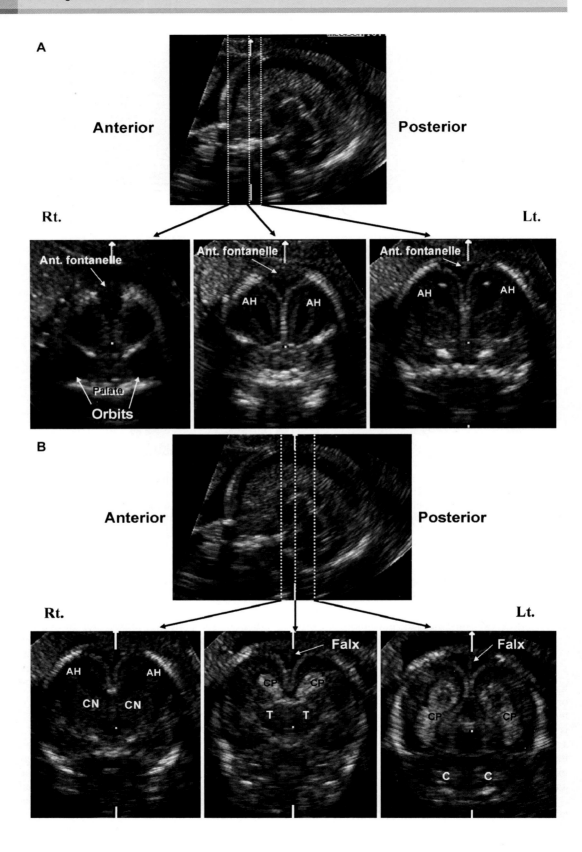

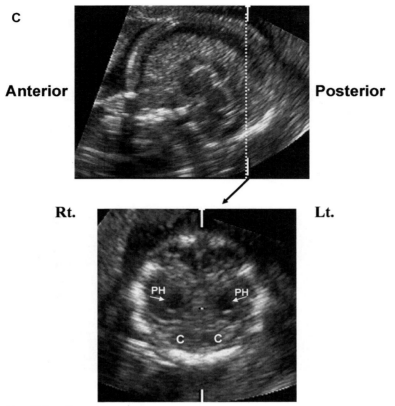

C

Anterior   Posterior

Rt.   Lt.

PH   PH

C   C

Fig. 12 (continued)

is impacted into the foramen magnum. If ventriculomegaly is present, the dangling choroid plexus can be also seen (see Fig. 21B). These abnormalities can be detected from the early second trimester of pregnancy. The lemon sign is present in virtually all cases between 16 and 24 postmenstrual weeks, but after 24 weeks of gestation, it is a less reliable marker because it is detected in only 13% to 50% of fetuses with spinal defects. The banana sign and the obliteration of the cisterna magna are present throughout gestation in 95% to 100% of fetuses with spinal dysraphism. However, after 24 postmenstrual weeks, cerebellar absence or inability to image the cerebellum is more common than the banana sign [7–12].

The presence of these sonographic clues (banana and lemon signs) should trigger a careful evaluation of the fetal spine. The spine should be examined in all three scanning planes. The sagittal view of the spine should include visualization of the skin covering the spine and the ossified vertebral body components. The findings on the sagittal plane may be irregularities of the bony spine, a bulge within the posterior contour of the fetal back, or an obvious disruption of the fetal skin contours [9]. During the second trimester of the pregnancy, the normal fetal spine, when viewed in an axial plane, has three ossification centers (a vertebral body and two lateral laminas), which form an enclosed triangular-shaped structure around the spinal cord. In cases of open spina bifida, this normal arrangement is lost and the two lateral laminas have a "U" shape and do not enclose the spinal cord and its membranes. The coronal section of the affected bony segment shows a divergent configuration replacing the normal parallel lines of the normal vertebral arches. Using 3D ultrasound, a volume of the fetal spine using the radiograph or maximum intensity mode would allow selective imaging of

Fig. 12. Transvaginal fetal neuroscan. Detailed targeted scan. For details see the corresponding text. (*A*) Three anterior coronal sections. (*B*) The midcoronal sections. (*C*) One posterior coronal section. (AH, anterior horn; C, cerebellum; CN, caudate nucleus; CP, choroid plexus; PH, posterior horn; T, thalamus.)

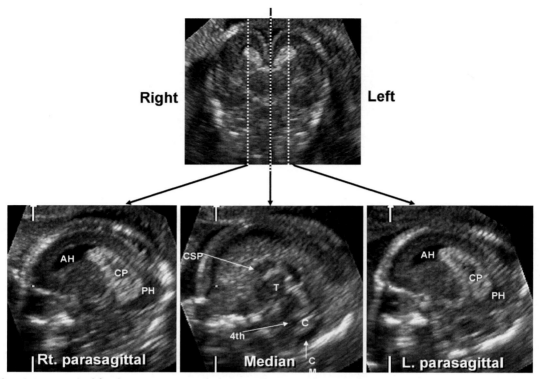

Fig. 13. Transvaginal fetal neuroscan. Detailed targeted scan. Right and left parasagittal (oblique) and a median plane are shown. Description of the structures is in the text. (AH, anterior horn; C, cerebellum; CP, choroid plexus; CSP, cavum septi pellucid; PH, posterior horn; T, thalamus.)

the bony spine and visualization of the bony spinal defect.

The constellation of indirect cranial findings (small posterior fossa, enlarged foramen magnum, downward herniation of cerebellar tonsils and vermis) and the direct spinal defect is termed the Arnold-Chiari type II malformation. This malformation is present in almost every case of thoracolumbar, lumbar, and lumbosacral myelomeningocele. In these cases, ventriculomegaly or hydrocephaly most likely is the result of a hindbrain malformation that blocks flow of cerebrospinal fluid through the fourth ventricle or posterior fossa, or from aqueductal stenosis, which is present in 40% to 75% of cases.

Spina bifida can be classified into three types: spina bifida aperta, or open spina bifida, in which the defect is not covered by skin (eg, myelomeningocele); spina bifida cystica, in which a mass is covered by skin (eg, meningocele); and spina bifida occulta, in which the spinal defect is covered by skin and no neural tissue is exposed or visible cystic mass evident [13,14]. Open spina bifida is associated with increased maternal serum α-feto protein and carries a worse prognosis, when compared

with the closed defect, spina bifida occulta, which has a good prognosis.

Agenesis of the corpus callosum

In ACC (Fig. 22), the basic examination not only would reveal the dilatation of the lateral ventricles (colpocephaly), and the abnormally shaped ventricle ("tear-shaped") (see Fig. 22C), but also the absence of the cavum septi pellucidi. However, if the fetal neurosonogram can be performed transvaginally, using 2D or 3D sonography, valuable information can be added to that obtained by the coronal and sagittal sections, which essentially solidifies the diagnosis of ACC. In the midcoronal transthalamic section, the lateral ventricles are usually widely separated and the interhemispheric fissure is seen reaching between the thalami and touching the third ventricle. In the median section, the lack of direct visualization of the corpus callosum establishes the diagnosis. In addition to the absent corpus callosum, the cingulate gyrus, which is normally present superior to it, is missing. The gyri and sulci rising above the roof of the third ventricle have a radiating appearance through the zone normally occupied by the cingulate gyrus. Also, in this

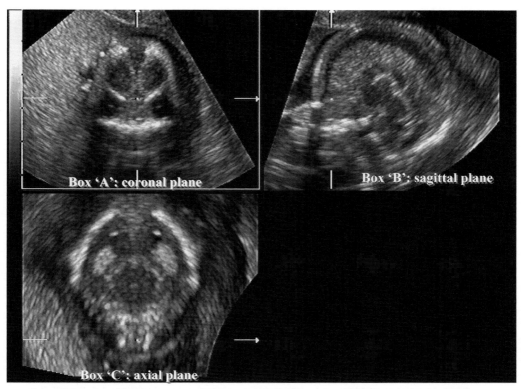

Fig. 14. Three-dimensional fetal neuroscan. This image describes the orthogonal planes (coronal, sagittal, and axial sections).

plane, using color or power Doppler reveals that the pericallosal artery is missing (see Fig. 22D, E).

In addition, complete ACC may include partial agenesis or hypoplasia of the corpus callosum. In cases of partial agenesis, the anterior portion (posterior genu and anterior body) is formed, but the posterior portion (posterior body and splenium) is not formed. The rostrum and the anterior/inferior genu are also not formed. Differentiating between hypogenesis, or a partial agenesis, and a normal corpus callosum can be difficult when relying on subjective assessment. Therefore, in this situation, the length, width, and thickness at the level of the anterior midbody of the corpus callosum can be measured and the measurement can be compared with published nomograms [15]. Also, identifying pericallosal artery along the length of the splenium of the corpus callosum may help. Differentiating hypoplasia of the corpus from a normal corpus callosum can be challenging because in hypoplasia it is fully formed but thinner than expected.

ACC occurs in at least 1 out of 4000 live births [16]. Up to one half of the cases of ACC may have other CNS anomalies such as lipomas,

interhemispheric cysts, Dandy-Walker continuum, gyral abnormalities, microcephaly, cephalocele, and meningocele. Approximately 10% of cases of callosal abnormalities have a chromosomal anomaly, and in the remaining 20% to 35%, a recognizable genetic syndrome may be present [17]. However, in cases of complete ACC, the number of recognizable syndromes drops to 10% to 15%; most cases do not have an identifiable cause [16].

Borderline ventriculomegaly

Borderline, or mild, ventriculomegaly is defined as the lateral ventricle measuring more than 10 mm but less than 12 mm in the absence of other CNS anomalies. In a significant number of cases, the ventriculomegaly is resolved during the course of the pregnancy. Several publications have reported that up to 90% of the fetuses having lateral ventricles of up to 12 mm demonstrated normal outcome. In approximately 4%, an abnormal karyotype may be present, of which trisomy 21 is the most common. In the absence of any other structural and karyotypic abnormalities, normal male fetuses are more likely to have lateral ventricles measuring more than 10 mm, when compared

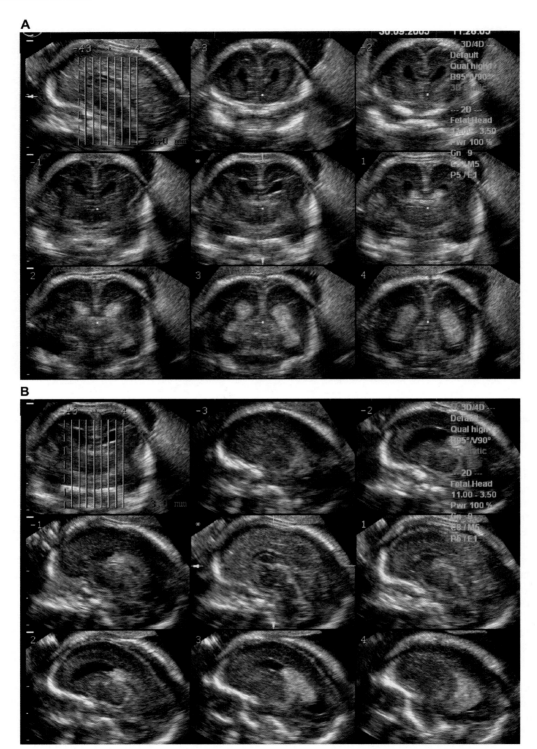

Fig. 15. Three-dimensional fetal neuroscan. Tomographic image displays. (A) Subsequent coronal planes. (B) Subsequent sagittal planes.

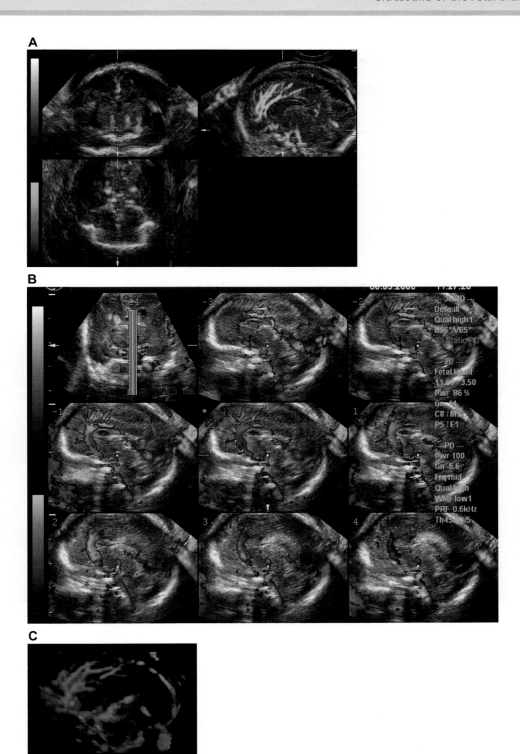

Fig. 16. Three-dimensional fetal neuroscan. Power Doppler angiogram of brain vessels. (*A*) Orthogonal display. (*B*) Consecutive sagittal sections. (*C*) Brain angiogram after the grayscale information was removed.

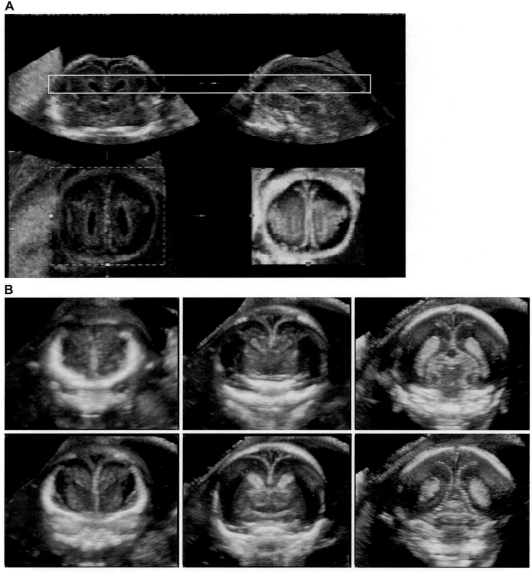

Fig. 17. Three-dimensional fetal neuroscan. (*A*) "Thick-slice" display within the rendering box (*lower right*). (*B*) Serial coronal sections depicted using "thick-slice" rendering.

with normal female fetuses of the same gestational age [18,19].

Enlarged cisterna magna

Another problem that can be detected during the basic examination is an enlarged cisterna magna measuring in excess of the upper normal limit of 10 mm. How do we evaluate this fetus?

1. Complete the basic examination of the head, assess the fetal spine, and perform a detailed anatomic survey of the fetus.

2. Obtain, if possible, the results of the first or second trimester maternal serum screen for aneuploidy or fetal karyotype.

3. Perform the fetal neurosonogram, with special emphasis on the posterior fossa.

In cases of large cisterna magna, the main differential diagnosis includes the Dandy-Walker continuum and arachnoid cysts.

The Dandy-Walker continuum

The posterior fossa abnormalities grouped in the Dandy-Walker continuum include Dandy-Walker

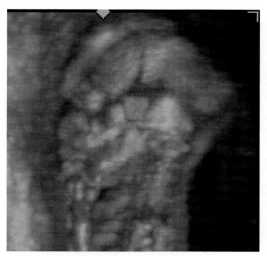

Fig. 18. Three-dimensional fetal neuroscan. Using the maximum mode, the skull bones are highlighted.

malformation (DWM), Dandy-Walker variant, Blake's pouch cyst, and mega-cisterna magna. During the basic examination using the transcerebellar plane, in addition to evaluating the size of the cisterna magna, the cerebellar hemispheres and the cerebellar vermis can be assessed. Septa in cisterna magna are commonly seen. It recently has been suggested that deviation from the normal appearance of the cisterna magna septa may be an early marker of abnormalities of the cerebellum, vermis, and brain stem. Therefore, in these cases, a targeted scan of the posterior fossa using multiplanar imaging is suggested [20]. In pregnancies of less than 20 weeks, obtaining an axial section that is too inferior may falsely give the impression of a vermian defect because the development of the cerebellar vermis occurs from a superior (rostral) to inferior (caudal) fashion and a normal connection between the fourth ventricle and cisterna magna cannot be demonstrated until the development of the vermis is complete [21–24]. Other findings that may be seen during the basic examination in cases of the Dandy-Walker spectrum include dilated lateral ventricles. In the transventricular plane, absent cavum septi pellucidi may be evident because DWM may be associated with ACC.

The next step in the assessment of a fetus with a large cisterna magna is the fetal neurosonogram, which, if possible, should be performed transvaginally using 2D or 3D sonography. When assessing posterior fossa abnormalities, the most important plane is the median plane. The region of the vermis

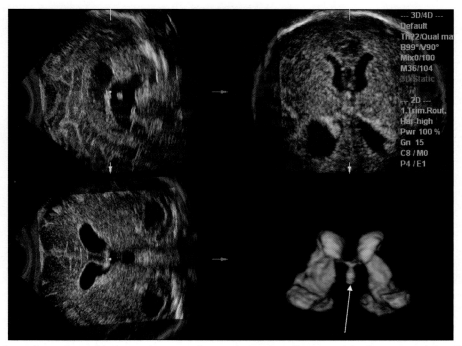

Fig. 19. Three-dimensional fetal neuroscan. In the rendering box (*lower right*), the "cast" of the fluid-filled lateral and third ventricles is demonstrated using the inversion rendering mode. Note the bilateral connection of the lateral ventricles to the third ventricle by way of the interventricular foramina (Monro).

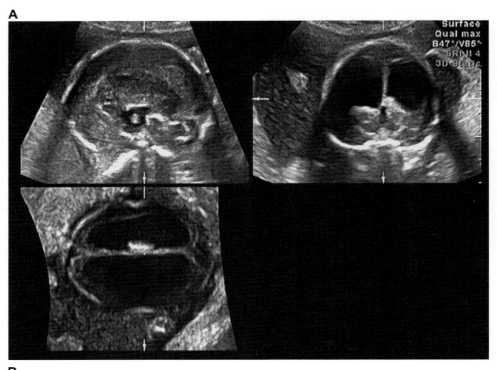

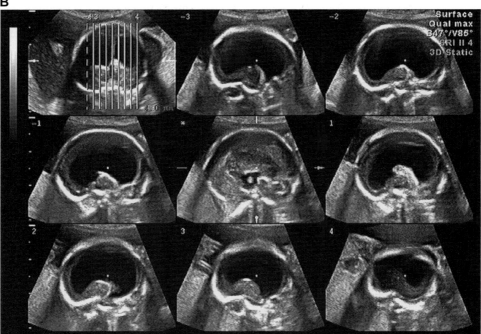

Fig. 20. Three-dimensional fetal neuroscan. (*A*) Orthogonal display. (*B*) Sagittal views. (*C*) Coronal sections. (*D*) Axial sections.

C

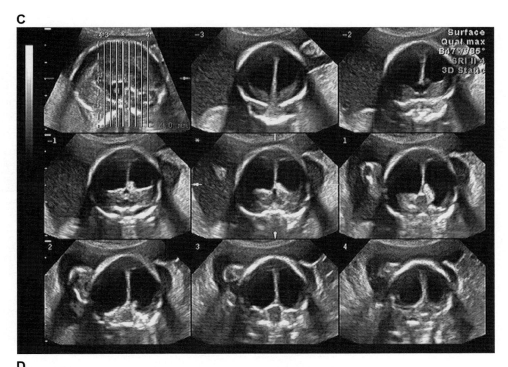

D

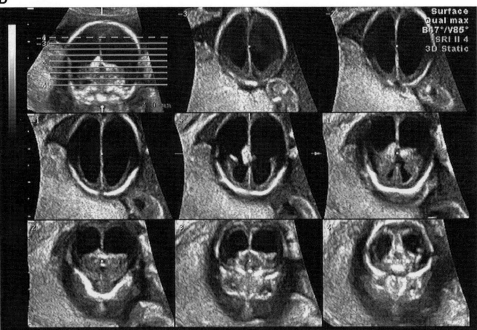

Fig. 20 (continued)

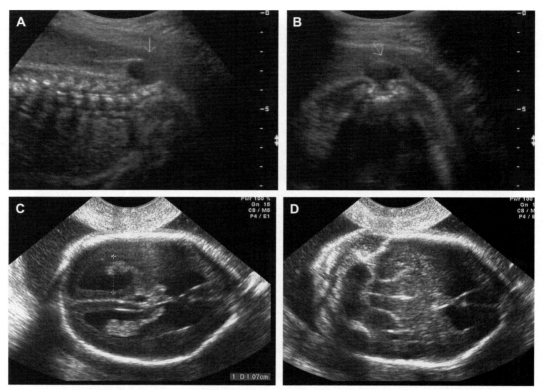

Fig. 21. Spina bifida and its effects on the fetal brain. (*A*) Sagittal section of the sacral spine with the lesion (*arrow*). (*B*) Axial section at the level of the sacral spine, showing the missing arch (*arrow*). (*C*) Ventriculomegaly and dangling choroid plexus. (*D*) The impacted cerebellum (banana) sign, and the temporal bone depression.

should be evaluated to determine if it is present, or completely or partially absent. Other information about the posterior fossa should also be obtained, including the existence of any communication between the fourth ventricle and the cisterna magna, and the position of the torcular Herophili. In cases of the classic DWM, the cerebellar vermis is absent, the fourth ventricle is dilated (communicating freely with the cisterna magna), and the torcular Herophili is elevated (Fig. 23A, B).

DWM is a relatively easy sonographic diagnosis to make in utero [25]. Notwithstanding the relative ease of diagnosis, only 60% to 80% of cases are detected antenatally. Recent improvements in the resolution of ultrasound equipment have led to the possibility of suspecting a DWM in the first trimester using transvaginal imaging [26].

DWM is a moderately rare malformation, occurring in 1 in 30,000 births. In 50% to 70% of cases, it is a severe anomaly with a list of associated brain anomalies. If isolated, the recurrence risk is 1% to 5%. In most survivors, a poor neurodevelopment is observed.

In cases of the Dandy-Walker variant, the inferior vermis is partially absent (Fig. 23C), but the torcular Herophili is not elevated. The Dandy-Walker variant is not as easy to diagnose in utero as the "full-blown" DWM. This condition involves variable hypoplasia or agenesis of the vermis, with or without enlargement of the cerebello-peduncular cistern, which communicates with the fourth ventricle. As previously mentioned, it can be over-diagnosed before 20 weeks' gestation, before complete vermian development.

Genetic factors may play a major role in the cause, and agenesis of the vermis is associated with a number of anomalies, such as (only the associated CNS findings are listed)

Aicardi's syndrome: ACC, with occasional ventriculomegaly, cortical heterotopias, choroid plexus papilloma

Chromosomal aneuploides: trisomy 8, trisomy 9, and triploidy

Fryns syndrome: ventriculomegaly, micrognathia

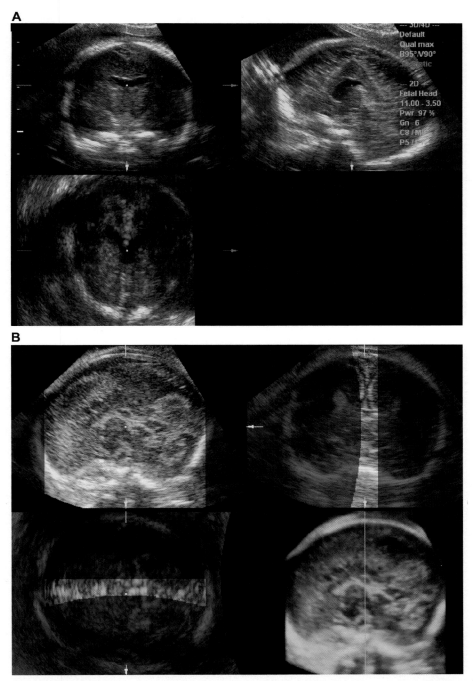

Fig. 22. Agenesis of corpus callosum. (*A*) Orthogonal planes. No corpus callosum is seen on the coronal (*upper left*) and sagittal section (*upper right*). (*B*) The "thick-slice" rendering (*lower right box*) demonstrates the lack of the corpus callosum. (*C*) Using the inversion mode shows the "cast" of the parallel lateral ventricles with the dilatation of the posterior horn (colpocephaly). (*D*) Power Doppler angiogram fails to demonstrate a pericallosal artery. (*E*) Serial gray scale and power Doppler angiogram of a case with ACC using the tomographic display.

C

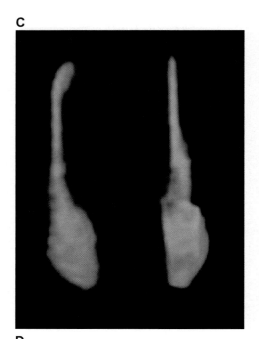

D

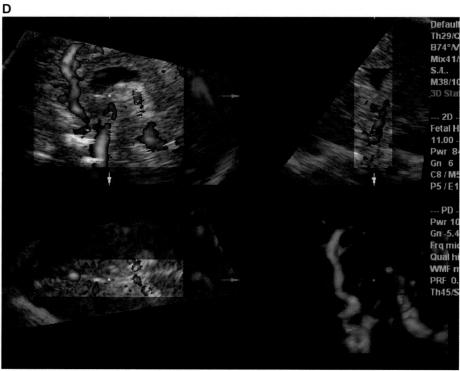

Fig. 22 (continued)

Meckel-Grubber syndrome: posterior encephalocele, ventriculomegaly, microcephaly

Neu-Laxova syndrome: microcephaly, dysgenesis of the corpus callosum, hypoplasia of the cerebellum, choroid plexus cysts, and lissencephaly

Smith-Lemli-Opitz syndrome: CNS findings include microcephaly, trigonocephaly, ACC, ventriculomegaly, cerebellar hypoplasia

Walker-Warburg syndrome: hydrocephaly, agyria, retinal dysplasia, and, at times, encephalocele [27–29].

E

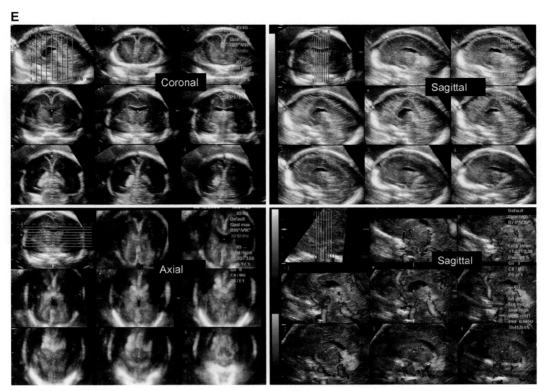

Coronal

Sagittal

Axial

Sagittal

Fig. 22 (*continued*)

The persistent Blake's Pouch cyst is not associated with any primary vermian hypoplasia or cerebellar dysplasia [20,30]. On the median plane, the cyst wall may be apparent (Fig. 24). The fluid inside the cyst is anechoic when compared with the slightly low-level echoic fluid in the surrounding subarachnoid space. The vermis may be displaced upward by the mass effect, which can also push the cerebellar hemispheres apart. This appearance is believed to be the result of failed fenestration laterally through the lateral aperture (Luschka) and in the median plane through the median aperture (Magendie), thereby preventing connection and fluid drainage between the so-created "cyst" and the subarachnoid space [30–34]. At times, ventriculomegaly can be seen as the result of the mass if it obliterates the cerebrospinal fluid drainage pathways. This entity is often first diagnosed in late adulthood. The prognosis is relatively good because postnatal shunting leads to re-expansion of the displaced brain structures.

In fetuses with mega-cisterna magna, the only finding is a cisterna magna (cerebellomedullary cistern) measuring greater than 10 mm, with a normal cerebellum, cerebellar vermis, and fourth ventricle (Fig. 25) [33,35]. Its clinical significance is uncertain and no clear-cut prognostic data are available. It can be totally asymptomatic but has been reported in association with other malformations or chromosomal aberrations.

Arachnoid cysts
In addition to the Dandy-Walker continuum, other conditions may account for an enlarged posterior fossa. In cases of posterior fossa arachnoid cysts, the basic examination transcerebellar plane reveals the enlarged posterior fossa. The cerebellum may be displaced as a result of the mass effect. In the median section, the cyst will be apparent and the cerebellum and fourth ventricle remain normal, although the tentorium may be slightly elevated and the vermis turned slightly upward. Approximately 5% to 10% of arachnoid cysts are located in the posterior fossa [31]. They have a relatively good prognosis, provided they are isolated and cause no pressure effect to result in ventriculomegaly.

Other central nervous system anomalies

Holoprosencephaly
The three types of holoprosencephaly are alobar, semilobar, and lobar. Of these, alobar and

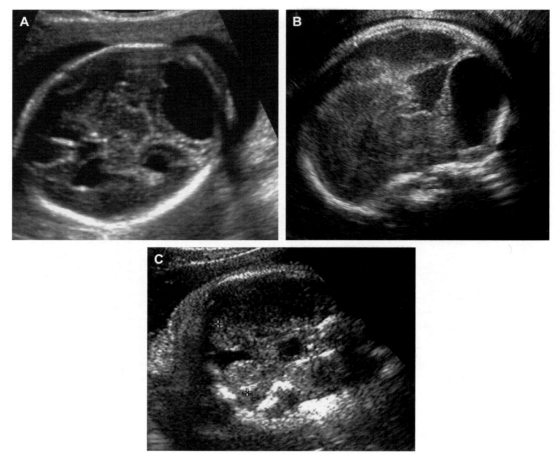

Fig. 23. The posterior fossa. (*A*) Axial section of a DWM. The splayed cerebellar hemispheres are seen. (*B*) Median section, demonstrating the elevated tentorium and torcular. (*C*) Dandy-Walker variant. Only the vermis is missing.

semilobar are relatively easy to diagnose. In alobar holoprosencephaly, the following structures are absent: interhemispheric fissure, falx cerebri, corpus callosum, and cavum septi pellucidi, and a single ventricle is present. The thalami are fused,

the third ventricle may be absent (Fig. 26), and various facial anomalies such as cyclopia, proboscis, and median clefts may be evident. Semilobar holoprosencephaly has the appearance of a single ventricle anteriorly; however, posteriorly the

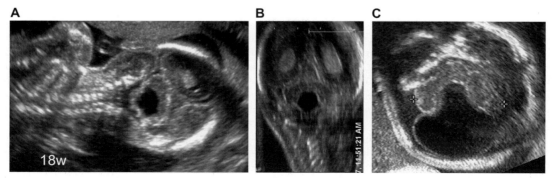

Fig. 24. Persistent Blake's pouch cyst. (*A,B*) Coronal sections. (*C*) Axial section, showing the cyst wall and the splayed cerebellar hemispheres.

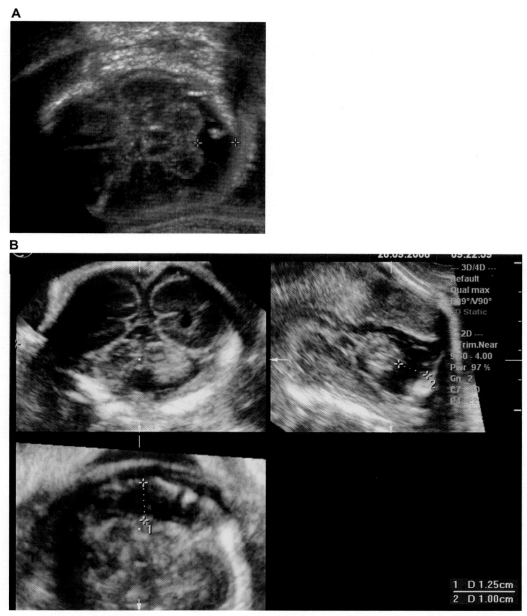

Fig. 25. Mega cistern magna. (*A*) Axial section. (*B*) 3D orthogonal planes: coronal (*upper left*), sagittal (*upper right*), and axial (*lower leftt*).

lateral ventricles appear separated, the cavum septi pellucidi is absent, and the corpus callosum is abnormal. Facial abnormalities may also be present, but are less severe than in the alobar type. Lobar holoprosencephaly has more subtle features. The corpus callosum is usually present (rarely it is hypoplastic or absent), the two lateral walls of the cavum septi pellucidi are absent, and the fornices are fused [36–38]. Its main differential diagnosis is septo-optic dysplasia. In septo-optic dysplasia, the lateral ventricles communicate with each other as the result of the absent cavum septi pellucidi, resulting in a box-shaped cavity below the corpus callosum. In addition, there is hypoplasia of the optic disk and the optic tracts. Using 3D, it is possible to image the optic chiasm; therefore, differentiating lobar holoprosencephaly from septo-optic dysplasia is technically possible [39]. Fetal MR

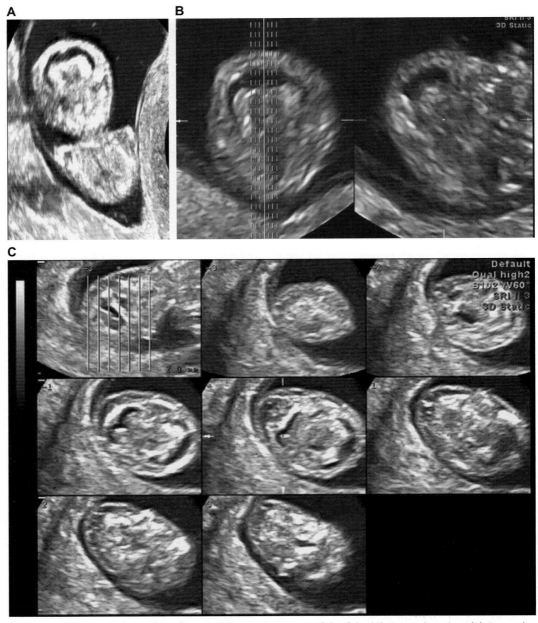

Fig. 26. Holoprosencephaly at 11 weeks. Note the total absence of the falx. (*A*) Coronal section. (*B*) Coronal and median sections. (*C*) Tomographic axial sections.

imaging may have a role in differentiating these two entities.

Hypoplastic cerebellum

Cerebellar hypoplasia may be unilateral (Fig. 27) or bilateral. It can be autosomal recessive [40] or X-linked, mapping to chromosomes Xq [41].

Rhombencephalosynapsis

Rhombencephalosynapsis is a rare vermian abnormality involving absence of the anterior vermis, a deficiency of the posterior vermis, and fusion of the cerebellar hemispheres (Fig. 28). The folia are oriented horizontally; the posterior fossa is small. Its cause is unknown and it occurs sporadically. Its severity and presentation correlate with

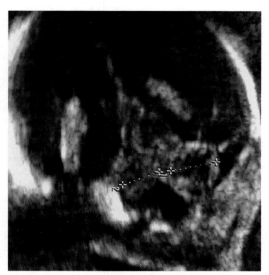

Fig. 27. Hemihypoplasia of the cerebellum. Note the asymmetric posterior fossa of the cerebellar hemispheres.

supratentorial anomalies. Most patients die early in life. Ultrasound diagnosis is easy and reliable [42].

Summary

Attention to the axial planes of the basic examination and coronal and sagittal planes of the fetal neuron-sonogram aid in the detection and characterization of fetal CNS anomalies.

References

[1] Monteagudo A, Timor-Tritsch IE. Development of fetal gyri, sulci and fissures: a transvaginal sonographic study. Ultrasound Obstet Gynecol 1997;9:222–8.

[2] Timor-Tritsch IE, Monteagudo A. Transvaginal sonographic evaluation of the fetal central nervous system. Obstet Gynecol Clin North Am 1991;18:713–48.

[3] International Society of Ultrasound in Obstetrics & Gynecology Education Committee. Sonographic examination of the fetal central nervous system: guidelines for performing the 'basic examination' and the 'fetal neurosonogram'. Ultrasound Obstet Gynecol 2007;29:109–16.

[4] Timor-Tritsch IE, Monteagudo A. Transvaginal fetal neurosonography: standardization of the planes and sections by anatomic landmarks. Ultrasound Obstet Gynecol 1996;8:42–7.

[5] Timor-Tritsch IE, Monteagudo A, Mayberry P. Three-dimensional ultrasound evaluation of the fetal brain: the three horn view. Ultrasound Obstet Gynecol 2000;16:302–6.

[6] Monteagudo A, Timor-Tritsch IE, Mayberry P. Three-dimensional transvaginal neurosonography of the fetal brain: 'navigating' in the volume scan. Ultrasound Obstet Gynecol 2000;16:307–13.

[7] Van den Hof MC, Nicolaides KH, Campbell J, et al. Evaluation of the lemon and banana signs in one hundred thirty fetuses with open spina bifida. Am J Obstet Gynecol 1990;162:322–7.

[8] Thiagarajah S, Henke J, Hogge WA, et al. Early diagnosis of spina bifida: the value of cranial ultrasound markers. Obstet Gynecol 1990;76:54–7.

[9] Pilu G, Romero R, Reece EA, et al. Subnormal cerebellum in fetuses with spina bifida. Am J Obstet Gynecol 1988;158:1052–6.

[10] Nyberg DA, Mack LA, Hirsch J, et al. Abnormalities of fetal cranial contour in sonographic detection of spina bifida: evaluation of the "lemon" sign. Radiology 1988;167:387–92.

[11] Campbell J, Gilbert WM, Nicolaides KH, et al. Ultrasound screening for spina bifida: cranial and cerebellar signs in a high-risk population. Obstet Gynecol 1987;70:247–50.

[12] Nicolaides KH, Campbell S, Gabbe SG, et al. Ultrasound screening for spina bifida: cranial and cerebellar signs. Lancet 1986;2:72–4.

[13] Botto LD, Moore CA, Khoury MJ, et al. Neural-tube defects. N Engl J Med 1999;341:1509–19.

[14] Byrd SE, Darling CF, McLone DG. Developmental disorders of the pediatric spine. Radiol Clin North Am 1991;29:711–52.

[15] Achiron R, Achiron A. Development of the human fetal corpus callosum: a high-resolution, cross-sectional sonographic study. Ultrasound Obstet Gynecol 2001;18:343–7.

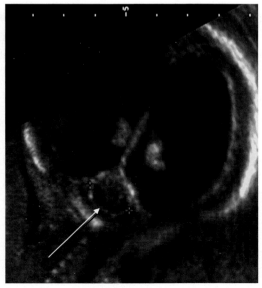

Fig. 28. Rhombencephalosynapsis, a rare anomaly of the posterior fossa. Note the undivided cerebellum in the shape of a ball (*arrow*).

[16] Paul LK, Brown WS, Adolphs R, et al. Agenesis of the corpus callosum: genetic, developmental and functional aspects of connectivity. Nat Rev Neurosci 2007;8:287–99.

[17] Bedeschi MF, Bonaglia MC, Grasso R, et al. Agenesis of the corpus callosum: clinical and genetic study in 63 young patients. Pediatr Neurol 2006;34:186–93.

[18] Gaglioti P, Danelon D, Bontempo S, et al. Fetal cerebral ventriculomegaly: outcome in 176 cases. Ultrasound Obstet Gynecol 2005;25:372–7.

[19] Signorelli M, Tiberti A, Valseriati D, et al. Width of the fetal lateral ventricular atrium between 10 and 12 mm: a simple variation of the norm? Ultrasound Obstet Gynecol 2004;23:14–8.

[20] Robinson AJ, Goldstein R. The cisterna magna septa: vestigial remnants of Blake's pouch and a potential new marker for normal development of the rhombencephalon. J Ultrasound Med 2007;26:83–95.

[21] Bromley B, Nadel AS, Pauker S, et al. Closure of the cerebellar vermis: evaluation with second trimester US. Radiology 1994;193:761–3.

[22] Malinger G, Ginath S, Lerman-Sagie T, et al. The fetal cerebellar vermis: normal development as shown by transvaginal ultrasound. Prenat Diagn 2001;21:687–92.

[23] Ben-Amin M, Perlitz Y, Peleg D. Transvaginal sonographic appearance of the cerebellar vermis at 14-16 weeks' gestation. Ultrasound Obstet Gynecol 2002;19:208–9.

[24] Babcook CJ, Chong BW, Salamat MS, et al. Sonographic anatomy of the developing cerebellum: normal embryology can resemble pathology. AJR Am J Roentgenol 1996;166:427–33.

[25] Klein O, Pierre-Kahn A, Boddaert N, et al. Dandy-Walker malformation: prenatal diagnosis and prognosis. Childs Nerv Syst 2003;19:484–9.

[26] Sherer DM, Shane H, Anyane-Yeboa K. First-trimester transvaginal ultrasonographic diagnosis of Dandy-Walker malformation. Am J Perinatol 2001;18:373–7.

[27] Low AS, Lee SL, Tan AS, et al. Difficulties with prenatal diagnosis of the Walker-Warburg syndrome. Acta Radiol 2005;46:645–51.

[28] Blin G, Rabbe A, Ansquer Y, et al. First-trimester ultrasound diagnosis in a recurrent case of Walker-Warburg syndrome. Ultrasound Obstet Gynecol 2005;26:297–9.

[29] Monteagudo A, Alayon A, Mayberry P. Walker-Warburg syndrome: case report and review of the literature. J Ultrasound Med 2001;20:419–26.

[30] Calabro F, Arcuri T, Jinkins JR. Blake's pouch cyst: an entity within the Dandy-Walker continuum. Neuroradiology 2000;42:290–5.

[31] Nelson MD Jr, Maher K, Gilles FH. A different approach to cysts of the posterior fossa. Pediatr Radiol 2004;34:720–32.

[32] Conti C, Lunardi P, Bozzao A, et al. Syringomyelia associated with hydrocephalus and Blake's pouch cyst: case report. Spine 2003;28:E279–83.

[33] Tortori-Donati P, Fondelli MP, Rossi A, et al. Cystic malformations of the posterior cranial fossa originating from a defect of the posterior membranous area. Mega cisterna magna and persisting Blake's pouch: two separate entities. Childs Nerv Syst 1996;12:303–8.

[34] Strand RD, Barnes PD, Poussaint TY, et al. Cystic retrocerebellar malformations: unification of the Dandy-Walker complex and the Blake's pouch cyst. Pediatr Radiol 1993;23:258–60.

[35] Barkovich AJ, Kjos BO, Norman D, et al. Revised classification of posterior fossa cysts and cystlike malformations based on the results of multiplanar MR imaging. AJR Am J Roentgenol 1989;153:1289–300.

[36] DeMyer W, Zeman W, Palmer CG. The face predicts the brain: diagnostic significance of medial facial anomalies for holoprosencephaly (arrhinencephaly). Pediatrics 1964;34:256–62.

[37] DeMyer W, Zeman W. Alobar holoprosencephaly (arhinencephaly) with median cleft lip and palate: clinical electroencephalographic and nosologic considerations. Confin Neurol 1963;23:1–36.

[38] Pilu G, Ambrosetto P, Sandri F, et al. Intraventricular fused fornices: a specific sign of fetal lobar holoprosencephaly. Ultrasound Obstet Gynecol 1994;4:65–7.

[39] Bault JP. Visualization of the fetal optic chiasma using three-dimensional ultrasound imaging. Ultrasound Obstet Gynecol 2006;28:862–4.

[40] Wichman A, Frank LM, Kelly TE. Autosomal recessive congenital cerebellar hypoplasia. Clin Genet 1985;27:373–82.

[41] Illarioshkin SN, Tanaka H, Markova ED, et al. X-linked nonprogressive congenital cerebellar hypoplasia: clinical description and mapping to chromosome Xq. Ann Neurol 1996;40:75–83.

[42] Utsunomiya H, Takano K, Ogasawara T, et al. Rhombencephalosynapsis: cerebellar embryogenesis. AJNR Am J Neuroradiol 1998;19:547–9.

ELSEVIER
SAUNDERS

ULTRASOUND
CLINICS

Ultrasound Clin 2 (2007) 245–263

Imaging of Fetal Tumors

Joao Fernando Kazan-Tannus, MD, PhD, Deborah Levine, MD*

The diagnosis of a fetal tumor is typically made at the time of a routine obstetric ultrasound or during a sonogram performed for enlarged fundal height in the case of a tumor associated with polyhydramnios. The anatomic region of the lesion suggests the involved organ, and thus the most likely tumor. Tissue characterization (cystic or solid, presence of calcifications, adjacent organ involvement) further narrows the differential diagnosis. Assessment with Doppler is important, because vascular tumors can lead to hydrops, and thus a worse prognosis. In select cases magnetic resonance (MR) imaging adds additional information. A complete description of the tumor is important in predicting outcome and in discussing the treatment options with the pregnant patient.

Neoplasms diagnosed up to 3 months after birth are considered congenital [1]. These congenital neoplasms account for 0.5% to 2% of all childhood neoplasms [2], with a prevalence of 1.7 to 13.5 per 100,000 live births [3]. This frequency does not account for those tumors in utero that lead to termination procedures or in utero demise [2].

The histologic type, incidence, and outcome of fetal neoplasms are different than those of the more general pediatric or even neonatal population. In addition, complications of neoplasms differ in the fetus and in the newborn in that hydrops can occur in utero. Assessment of tumor involvement in the airway is important before delivery, because delivery by the ex utero intrapartum treatment procedure (EXIT) can be lifesaving [4].

Once a tumor is diagnosed, sonographic follow-up is important. Often a tumor grows more slowly than the fetus overall, and thus the relative mass effect of the tumor decreases during gestation. Even a benign mass, however, if large enough or very vascular, can lead to cardiac failure and hydrops. Tumors can also lead to fetal malposition, dystocia, and need for delivery by cesarean section.

In this review the authors illustrate various fetal tumors and suggest how prenatal imaging can improve counseling and management of these patients.

Intracranial tumors

True neoplasms

Fetal intracranial tumors tend to be supratentorial (up to 79% [5]), as compared with pediatric

Department of Radiology, Beth Israel Deaconess Medical Center, 330 Brookline Avenue, Boston, MA 02215, USA
* Corresponding author.
E-mail address: dlevine@bidmc.harvard.edu (D. Levine).

doi:10.1016/j.cult.2007.07.007

intracranial tumors, of which most are infratentorial [6]. These tumors can cause enlargement of the fetal head because of the tumor itself, hemorrhage, or ventricular obstruction and hydrocephalus. When a lesion is visualized in the brain, it is important to differentiate a neoplasm from a hematoma. Hemorrhage in the brain may appear as a heterogeneous intracranial mass. Doppler analysis can be helpful in these cases, because a hematoma does not show flow, whereas a tumor typically demonstrates increased vascularity. It is important to recognize, however, that brain tumors frequently bleed, leading to a confusing sonographic appearance. With a brain hemorrhage or a brain neoplasm, the enlarged head can lead to dystocia, necessitating cesarean delivery [7–9]. Once a brain lesion is diagnosed, follow-up for assessing fetal growth and head size is therefore important in determining the timing and mode of delivery.

The most common intracranial tumor is the teratoma, comprising up to one half of all fetal intracranial tumors [3]. These lesions have a poor prognosis, with most fetuses dying in utero or shortly after birth [7,10]. The tumors tend to be midline, to exhibit rapid growth, are heterogeneous in echo texture, and may have regions of calcification.

The second most common fetal intracranial tumor is the astrocytoma. This also has a poor prognosis, with an overall survival rate of approximately 30% [10]. As expected from their histology, low-grade astrocytomas have a better prognosis than do higher-grade tumors [11]. Low-grade lesions present as a solid supratentorial mass. Grade IV astrocytomas (glioblastoma multiforme) are uncommon, comprising 18% of fetal intracranial tumors [7,8]. Glioblastoma (Fig. 1) [12] appears as a large supratentorial heterogeneous hyperechoic mass occupying most of one hemisphere, sometimes with midline shift and obstructive hydrocephalus [7,8,13]. The tumors grow rapidly, with high rates of hemorrhage [14,15]. Congestive heart failure may occur secondary to the hypervascularity of the tumor [9,16]. Visualization of a vertical disconjugate gaze in coronal views indicates brain stem involvement and poor postnatal prognosis [17].

Primitive neuroectodermal tumors are less common (13%) and have a poor prognosis (88% fatal) [7,10]. Other uncommon tumors include lipomas and choroid plexus papillomas that have better prognosis than the previously mentioned tumors [7,8,18]. Intracranial lipomas are well-defined, hyperechoic lesions that tend to be midline and may be associated with callosal dysgenesis. Choroid plexus papillomas are well-defined, lobulated hyperechoic intraventricular masses that may cause ventricular obstruction and hydrocephalus.

Rare fetal intracranial tumors include medulloepithelioma (mesencephalon and cerebellum are the primary sites, highly aggressive tumor that invades local structures and spreads along the cerebrospinal fluid pathways [19]), craniopharyngioma (arise from 'Rathke pouch, present as a calcified cystic suprasellar mass causing macrocephaly, similar in appearance to teratoma [20,21]), meningioma (half arise from the parietal or occipital meninges and half are malignant [22,23]), ganglioglioma (vary in size and are well-circumscribed with finely granular and calcifications [24]), and ependymoma (arise from the region of the fourth ventricle presenting with macrocephaly and hydrocephalus [25,26]).

Subependymal nodules in tuberous sclerosis

Although not true neoplasms, subependymal nodules are included in this review because they can present as obstructing lesions, simulating a brain tumor [27,28]. These lesions are typically not visualized with ultrasound unless they are large enough to cause obstruction. The subependymal nodules can be seen by MR imaging as early as 20 weeks gestational age [29,30]. If tuberous sclerosis complex is suspected based on family history or the presence of cardiac rhabdomyomas, fetal MR imaging can be helpful in establishing the diagnosis (Fig. 2) [31]. On MR imaging, using T2-weighted imaging (T2WI) with single shot fast-spin echo (SSFSE), these subependymal nodules are low signal intensity lesions that line and project into the ventricles. On T1-weighted imaging (T1WI) they are of high signal intensity. Cortical tubers can also be present and are also visualized as low signal intensity on T2WI and high signal intensity on T1WI. It is expected that a combination of ultrasound (assessing for cardiac rhabdomyomas) and MR imaging (assessing for intracranial involvement) will lead to improved prenatal diagnosis of tuberous sclerosis [29].

Scalp lesions

If a scalp mass is found, the differential diagnosis includes encephalocele, epidermal/dermal cyst, lipoma, hematoma, protruding pacchionian granulations, cystic hygroma, and hemangioma [32–34]. Many of these are benign lesions and not true neoplasms. Because encephaloceles can have a poor prognosis, however, it is of utmost importance to carefully assess the skull and brain underlying the scalp lesion. Occipital encephaloceles are most common, representing 80% of cases. The α-fetoprotein is typically elevated but may be normal if the lesion is entirely covered by skin [32]. If the fetus is in cephalic position, a vaginal scan

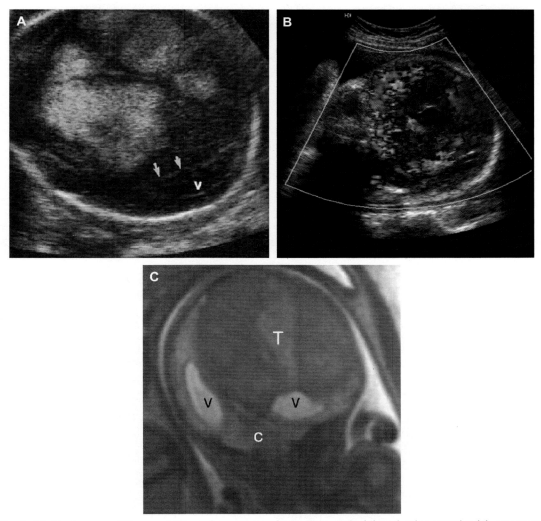

Fig. 1. Glioblastoma multiforme at 33 weeks gestational age. Gray scale (*A*) and color Doppler (*B*) sonograms demonstrate an enlarged head (with head size 7 weeks greater than expected for dates) with multifocal echogenic hypervascular intracranial masses that replace most of the parenchyma and displace the falx and lateral ventricles (*C*). Coronal T2-weighted image shows the heterogeneous tumor (*T*), which displaces the falx and lateral ventricles (*v*). Note the compressed cerebellum (*c*). The diffuse heterogeneity of the process is most consistent with an aggressive neoplasm, such as glioblastoma multiforme, rather than a diffuse vascular malformation. Glioblastoma multiforme was confirmed at autopsy. Prenatal imaging in this case allowed for the decision to be made before delivery to not admit the infant to the intensive care unit and to not resuscitate the infant at birth. (*A,B*) *Reproduced from* Morof DF, Levine D, Stringer KF, et al. Congenital glioblastoma multiforme: prenatal diagnosis on the basis of sonography and magnetic resonance imaging. J Ultrasound Med 2001;20(12):1369–75; with permission.)

can be helpful to further assess the skull and intracranial contents. In cases in which the diagnosis of a scalp mass is unclear by ultrasound, MR imaging can be helpful in showing the normal underlying brain.

Epidermal cysts are generally hypoechoic. They are covered by skin and have no neural involvement [32].

Scalp hemangiomas (Fig. 3) [35] are heterogeneous vascular masses in close contact to the bone [36–38]. Doppler ultrasound may show blood flow, which differentiates this type of mass from the other more cystic scalp lesions. Hemangiomas often form an obtuse angle with the adjacent skull, whereas encephaloceles more typically form an acute angle [39–41].

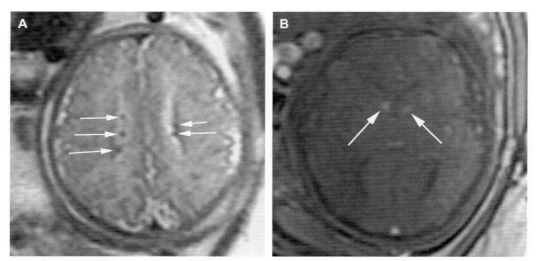

Fig. 2. Screening for tuberous sclerosis in a fetus with cardiac rhabdomyomas at 34 weeks gestational age. (*A*) Axial T2-weighted image shows low signal intensity subependymal nodules (*arrows*). (*B*) Axial T1-weighted image at a slightly lower level shows the nodules to be of high signal intensity. The brain findings were only seen on MR imaging. (*Reproduced from* Levine D, Barnes P. MR imaging of fetal CNS abnormalities. In: Levine D, editor. Atlas of fetal MRI. 1st edition. Boca Raton (FL): Taylor & Francis Group; 2005; with permission. Copyright © 2005, Routlege/Taylor & Francis Group, LLC.)

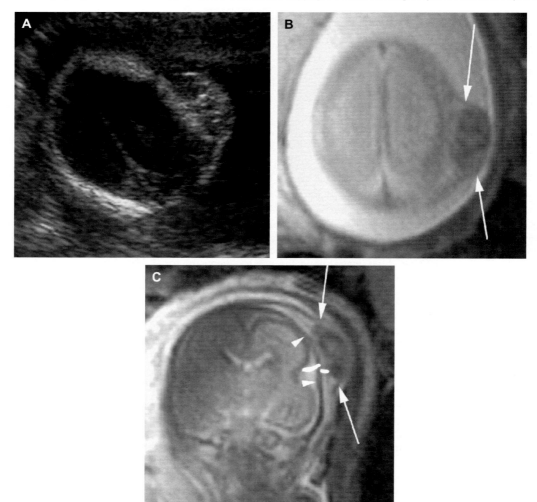

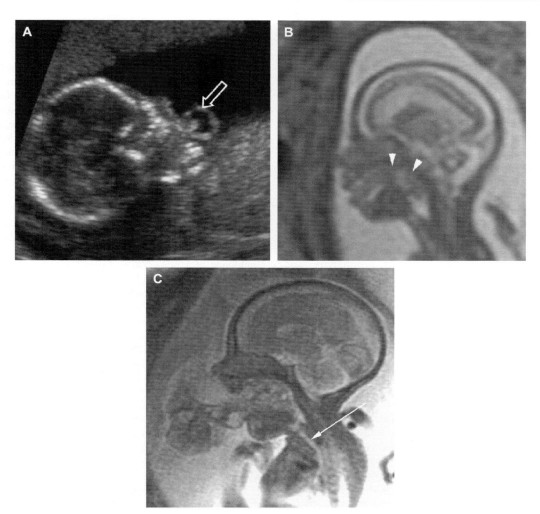

Fig. 4. Oropharyngeal teratoma. (*A*) Oblique sagittal sonogram at 16 weeks gestational age of the face shows an exophytic soft-tissue mass (*open arrow*). (*B*) Sagittal T2-weighted image at 16 weeks gestational age shows the soft-tissue mass (*arrowheads*) filling the oropharynx. (*C*) Sagittal T2-weighted image at 28 weeks gestational age shows a lobulated mass with cystic and solid components that distends the mouth. A patent trachea in the mid and lower neck was demonstrated (*arrow*). This information (and information about a nuchal cord that also went around the fetal shoulder in a subsequent MR imaging examination, not shown) was important to planning delivery by EXIT procedure for tracheostomy placement. The mass was surgically removed on day 1 of life, and reconstruction of the mandible was successful. (*A,B*) *Reproduced from* Morof D, Levine D, Grable I, et al. Oropharyngeal teratoma: prenatal diagnosis and assessment using sonography, MRI, and CT with management by ex utero intrapartum treatment procedure. AJR Am J Roentgenol 2004;183(2):493–6; with permission.)

Fig. 3. Scalp hemangioma at 22 weeks gestational age. (*A*) Transverse sonogram shows a scalp mass with flattening of the calvarium. No bony defect was visualized; however, there were regions in which the entire bone could not be visualized. Axial (*B*) and coronal (*C*) T2-weighted images show skin thickening with a low signal intensity mass (*arrows*) protruding from the soft tissues of the scalp external to the skull (*arrowheads*). The mass does not involve intracranial contents. MR imaging clarified that this was a scalp hemangioma and not an encephalocele, and the patient decided to continue the pregnancy. (*B,C*) *From* Levine D. Compendium of fetal MRI. Available at: bidmc.harvard.edu/content/bidmc/departments/radiology/files/fetalatlas/default. htm; with permission.

Tumors of the scalp and face

Tumors of the scalp and face are important to carefully characterize with respect to size, tissue characteristics, and potential brain and airway involvement. They are commonly teratomas and less commonly lymphangiomas or hemangiomas [42]. In cases in which sonography has not adequately demonstrated the airway, MR imaging can be helpful. In cases in which the airway is potentially compromised from a facial or neck tumor, delivery by the EXIT procedure can be lifesaving [4,9,43,44].

Oropharyngeal teratoma (Fig. 4), also known as an epignathus, has an incidence of 1:35,000 to 1:200,000 live births [45]. The sonographic findings include a heterogeneous mass with or without calcifications originating in the oropharynx and potentially extending out of the mouth. At times these lesions invade the skull, therefore assessment for intracranial involvement is extremely important, because this dramatically worsens the outcome [46,47]. Polyhydramnios occurs in approximately one third of cases [48]. Cesarean section may be necessary because of large tumor size [49] or because of positional deformity of the fetus [50].

A less common tumor of the fetal face and neck is the hemangioma. Similar to other locations, this vascular tumor may be associated with high output cardiac failure because of blood shunting or because of the Kasabach-Merrit sequence with severe consumption of blood cells by the tumor leading to hemolytic anemia [51,52]. In such cases, the lesion is seen to have dilated vessels with low resistance flow, indicating arteriovenous communications.

Solid head lesions may be due to a rhabdomyoma, rhabdomyosarcoma, or teratoma. Sonographically these are typically undistinguishable, although heterogeneity of echogenicity and calcifications would suggest a teratoma [53,54]. Rare fetal facial tumors include gingival granular cell tumor or congenital epulis (benign tumor that originates from the alveolar ridge and sonographically appears as a solid mass protruding from the mouth [42,55]) and retinoblastoma (originating from the retina during the first differentiation of the pars optica, prenatally appearing as an irregular echogenic oval-shaped tumor protruding from the eye socket [56]).

Neck

Lymphangiomas (Fig. 5) [57], teratomas (Fig. 6) [57], and hemangiomas can occur in the neck region. In the anterior neck, other masses can be caused by soft-tissue lesions, such as sarcomas, hamartomas (as can be seen in rare cases of tuberous sclerosis [58]), or fetal goiter. Masses in the anterior neck may cause hyperextension of the neck when large and are frequently associated with polyhydramnios [59,60].

Lymphangiomas are congenital lymphatic malformations that are caused by aberrations in normal lymphatic development. Lymphangiomas can be classified into three groups: (1) lymphangioma simplex, consisting of capillary-sized channels, (2) cavernous lymphangioma, consisting of dilated lymphatic channels frequently with a fibrous adventitial covering, and (3) cystic lymphangiomas or hygromas, composed of multiple cysts of varying size lined by endothelial cells [61,62]. Although lymphangiomas are not technically neoplastic, they are included in this article, because they overlap in appearance with other neoplasms. Lymphangiomas occur commonly in the neck, with an incidence of 1 per 6000 pregnancies, generally in the posterior triangle [60]. When the jugular lymph sacs fail to drain normally, they distend and form septated structures [63–65]. Progression to hydrops (and demise) can occur [64,65]. They may grow rapidly, compromising fetal growth or extending into the neck and obstructing the fetal airway [59,60,63]. Clinical presentation depends on the site of involvement and compression to adjacent organs.

On sonography, lymphangiomas typically present as multilocular cystic masses with thin septations. Scattered low-level echoes, a solid component, or fluid-fluid levels caused by bleeding and fibrin deposition can occur (see Fig. 5) [57]. The border of a lymphangioma can be indistinct with diffuse infiltration into surrounding soft tissues [66,67].

When these occur in the region of the oropharynx, it is important to assess involvement of the base of the tongue, because tongue lesions can interfere with handling of secretions and ability to breastfeed. Unlike teratomas or other vascular tumors, lymphangiomas do not have prominent blood vessels [68]. MR imaging may elucidate extension to the base of the tongue, which is a difficult area to assess with ultrasound. In addition, MR imaging can show the overall extent of large tumors when the field of view by ultrasound limits this assessment [69].

It may be difficult to distinguish a hemangioma from a lymphangioma, because both tumor types have heterogeneous echotexture with cystic and solid components. Doppler can be useful in those situations, showing prominent vascularity in hemangiomas.

Goiter is not a neoplasm but can be suggested when there are bilateral, echogenic, symmetric, bilobed masses in the region of the thyroid [70]. Goiter can have high vascular flow, leading to cardiac failure [70]. The intra-amniotic administration of thyroid hormone can be used to reduce the goiter size and subsequently its affect on the fetal circulation [70–72].

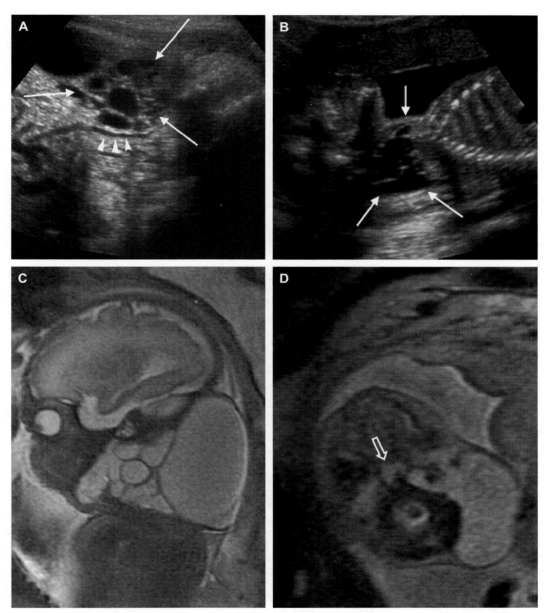

Fig. 5. Cervical lymphangioma at 34 weeks gestational age. Coronal (*A*) and sagittal (*B*) sonograms show a left neck septated cystic mass (*arrows*) extending to midline and deviating the trachea (*arrowheads*). Sagittal (*C*) and axial (*D*) T2-weighted images show the mass extending to the base of the tongue (without direct involvement of the tongue) and extending to the oropharynx, but the oropharynx is still midline (*open arrow*). MR imaging demonstrating the lack of obstruction of the oropharyngeal airway allowed for delivery by cesarean section instead of EXIT procedure (*C*). (*Reproduced from* Levine D, Stroustrup Smith A. MR imaging of the fetal skull, face, and neck. In: Levine D, editor. Atlas of fetal MRI. 1st edition. Boca Raton (FL): Taylor & Francis Group; 2005; with permission. Copyright © 2005, Routlege/Taylor & Francis Group, LLC.)

Thorax

Lymphangiomas (Fig. 7) [73] can be found in any part of the chest, with similar sonographic findings as those described in the previous section, being a thin-walled, multiseptate, asymmetric, fluid-filled mass [74]. The variability of the imaging findings is caused by the amount of tissue (connective tissue, muscle tissue, adipose tissue) and necrosis of the cysts [75]. Doppler does not show aberrant vascularity [59].

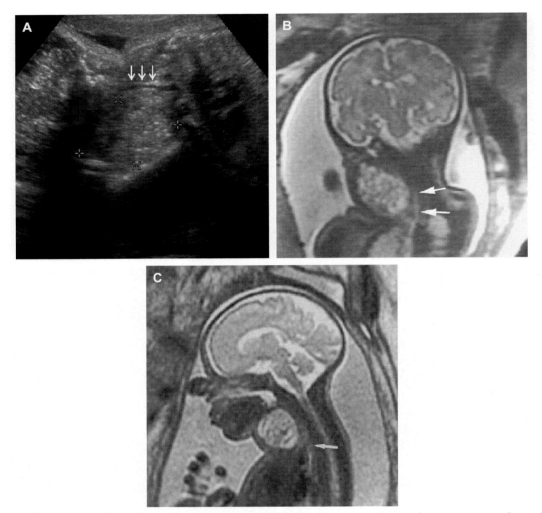

Fig. 6. Thyroid teratoma at 28 weeks gestational age. (*A*) Sagittal sonogram shows a heterogeneous echogenic mass (*calipers*) that deviates the trachea (*arrows*) posteriorly. Coronal (*B*) and sagittal (*C*) T2-weighted images show a heterogeneous cystic and solid neck mass extending from the base of the tongue on the right, continuing just above the thoracic inlet. The trachea (*arrows*) is deviated by the mass. The airway is visualized above and below the mass on the sagittal view, but at the most posterior mid aspect of the mass it is poorly visualized. The EXIT procedure was required in this case, and the neonate was intubated before clamping the umbilical cord (*C*). (*Reproduced from* Levine D, Stroustrup Smith A. MR imaging of the fetal skull, face, and neck. In: Levine D, eitor. Atlas of fetal MRI. 1st edition. Boca Raton (FL): Taylor & Francis Group; 2005; with permission. Copyright © 2005, Routlege/Taylor & Francis Group, LLC.)

In the anterior chest, the fetal thymus (Fig. 8) can appear as a mass. Knowledge of the normal appearance of the thymus is important to not mistake this normal structure for a neoplasm.

Mediastinal teratomas (Fig. 9) [73] have rarely been discovered during the prenatal period. These are visualized as multilobulated cystic and solid masses, sometimes with calcifications [76]. When large, these tumors can cause respiratory distress or hydrops [77]. MR imaging can be used for accurate measurement of lung volumes for prediction of pulmonary hypoplasia [78]. The conspicuity of the signal intensity in fetal lung is high enough that, even in large chest masses, small amounts of compressed normal lung can be visualized.

Pericardial teratomas typically arise from the great vessels [79] and may be massive [80]. The lesion is typically echogenic, mixed cyst and solid, sometimes containing calcifications. Associated pericardial effusion can lead to tamponade [80,81].

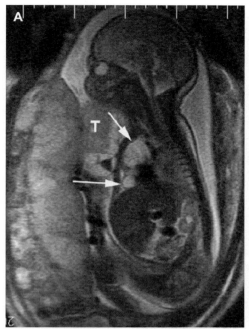

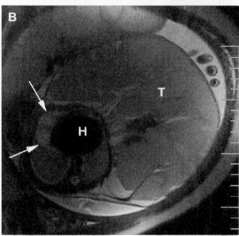

Fig. 7. Mediastinal lymphangioma at 26 weeks gestational age. Sagittal (*A*) and axial (*B*) T2-weighted images show the large tumor (*T*) with intrathoracic extent (*arrows*) seen as regions of high signal intensity in the anterior mediastinum. MR imaging volumetry (not shown) demonstrated that the volume of the tumor was 1.5 times that of the fetus. The impact of MR imaging in this case was the clear delineation of the tumor size and extent, which allowed for improved parental counseling. H, heart.

The most common cardiac tumor is the rhabdomyoma (Fig. 10). These lesions are seen as echogenic masses in the heart. As mentioned, these can be seen in association with tuberous sclerosis complex, with the intracranial lesions being better detected on MR imaging. Sixty percent of infants who have

tuberous sclerosis have cardiac rhabdomyomas [47,82]. These lesions can be detected as early as 19 weeks gestational age [83,84]. If one rhabdomyoma is present, the likelihood of tuberous sclerosis complex is 50% [47]. If two or more of these lesions are present, the likelihood of the complex is 80% to 100% [47].

Cardiac myxoma is a rare entity in fetal diagnosis [47]. The sonographic and clinical findings are based on the affected chamber or conduction disturbances [47].

When a cardiac tumor is visualized, a formal fetal echocardiogram is recommended to assess for any outflow obstruction. The location of the tumor, associated arrhythmias, and hydrops determines the outcome more than solely the histologic type [85–87]. For example, rhabdomyomas may cause outflow obstruction and lead to hydrops fetalis and in utero demise. In other cases, even large intracardiac lesions if they do not obstruct flow can be asymptomatic.

Hepatic tumors

Hepatic hemangiomata (Fig. 11) are among the most common tumors of the liver diagnosed during fetal and neonatal life, infancy, and childhood [88,89]. They are seen as well-circumscribed abdominal masses that may be small or large, up to 10 cm [66,88–92]. Hemangioma may be solitary or multiple, the latter sometimes forming part of the much less common generalized hemangiomatosis syndrome [89,93].

Hemangioendothelioma (Fig. 12) is a lesion composed of large endothelial-lined vascular channels, which is histologically distinct from hemangioma [3]. If a hepatic mass is purely hypoechoic, it is probably a hemangioendothelioma rather than a hemangioma [88,94]. It is important to describe the Doppler findings of location, size, diameter, and number of vessels, and vascular shunts. Draining veins will have high velocity, low pulsatility blood flow compared with the other intrahepatic vessels [89].

Congenital hepatic hemangiomas and hemangioendotheliomas typically regress in the first 2 years of life [95]. Although these lesions are benign they may cause life-threatening complications because of high-output cardiac failure or consumptive coagulopathy (Kasabach-Merrit sequence) and hepatic rupture [88,96–98]. If signs of high output cardiac failure are present, the lesions can be treated in utero with maternal corticosteroids leading to regression of the lesion [99,100]. Percutaneous umbilical cord sampling and transfusion can be helpful in cases with anemia [89].

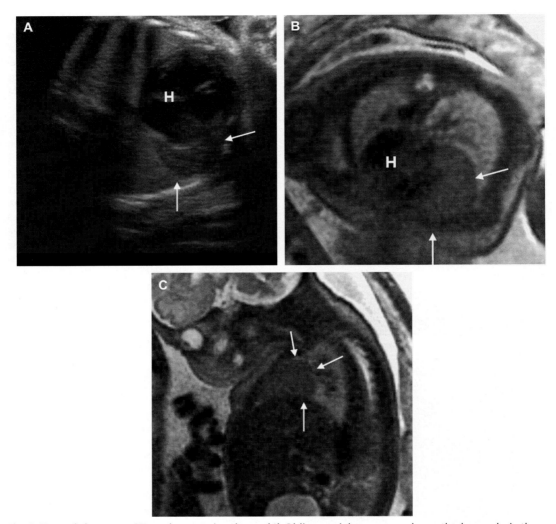

Fig. 8. Normal thymus at 37 weeks gestational age. (*A*) Oblique axial sonogram shows the hypoechoic thymus (*arrows*) adjacent to the heart (*H*). Axial (*B*) and sagittal (*C*) T2-weighted images show the thymus (*arrows*) with low signal intensity in relation to the lungs. The heart (*H*) is not deviated by the thymus.

Other less common hepatic masses are hamartomas (generally cystic septated masses [101]), adenoma (solid echogenic masses [102,103]), hepatoblastoma (heterogeneous solid vascular mass [104,105]), and metastases (generally from neuroblastoma).

Adrenal neoplasms

When a fetal suprarenal lesion is visualized, the differential diagnosis includes adrenal hemorrhage, infradiaphragmatic sequestration, and neuroblastoma.

Fetal neuroblastoma (**Fig. 13**) is usually detected in the third trimester of pregnancy [106]. It may be solid, cystic, or hemorrhagic with cystic and solid

components [106–109]. High catecholamine levels may lead to hydrops, maternal hypertension, or pre-eclampsia [109]. As mentioned, neuroblastoma can metastasize to the liver [104]. Fetal neuroblastoma has a much better outcome than pediatric neuroblastoma [3,110]. The tumors frequently regress in utero or in the neonatal period.

The causes of adrenal hemorrhage include stress, trauma at birth, hypoxia, thrombocytopenia, septicemia, and congenital syphilis [107,111]. In the acute stage, adrenal hemorrhage appears solid and echogenic, becoming hypoechoic as liquefaction occurs and appearing anechoic as the process resolves [107]. It may be impossible to differentiate an adrenal hemorrhage from a hemorrhagic neuroblastoma. Over time the internal

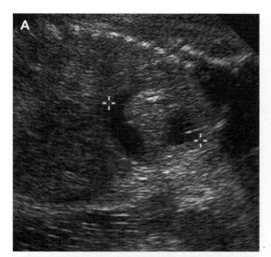

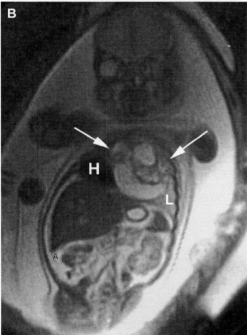

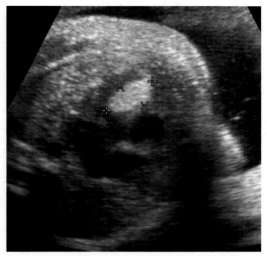

Fig. 10. Cardiac rhabdomyoma at 30 weeks gestational age. Axial sonogram of the heart shows an echogenic mass (*calipers*) consistent with a cardiac rhabdomyoma. Other images showed multiple other smaller rhabdomyomas. This finding of multiple cardiac rhabdomyomas puts the patient at extremely high risk for tuberous sclerosis.

flow is not visualized within an adrenal hemorrhage [108].

An important lesion in the differential diagnosis of a suprarenal mass is the extrapulmonary sequestration. This is visualized as an echogenic mass, typically on the left side [106]. These are visualized earlier in gestation than are neuroblastomas, which

Fig. 9. Mediastinal teratoma at 29 weeks gestational age. (*A*) Coronal sonogram shows a heterogeneous mixed echogenicity mass in the anterior thorax. (*B*) Coronal T2-weighted image shows the heterogenous mediastinal mass (*arrows*) deviating the heart (*H*) inferiorly and to the right. Note ascites in the abdomen. L, left lung (*B*). (*Reproduced from* Levine D. MR of fetal thoracic abnormalities. In Levine D, editor. Atlas of fetal MRI. 1st edition. Boca Raton (FL): Taylor & Francis Group; 2005; with permission. Copyright © 2005, Routlege/Taylor & Francis Group, LLC.)

characteristics of adrenal hemorrhage change as the blood clot evolves. The region of hemorrhage also eventually reduces in size and the wall may calcify [106–109,112]. Unlike neuroblastoma,

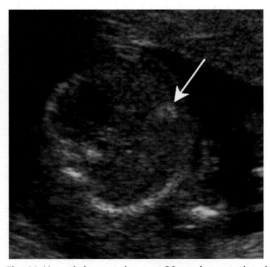

Fig. 11. Hepatic hemangioma at 20 weeks gestational age. Transverse sonogram shows a small homogeneous echogenic liver mass (*arrow*) characteristic of a hepatic hemangioma. Doppler (not shown) showed no increase in vascularity. This type of lesion is unlikely to cause problems in pregnancy.

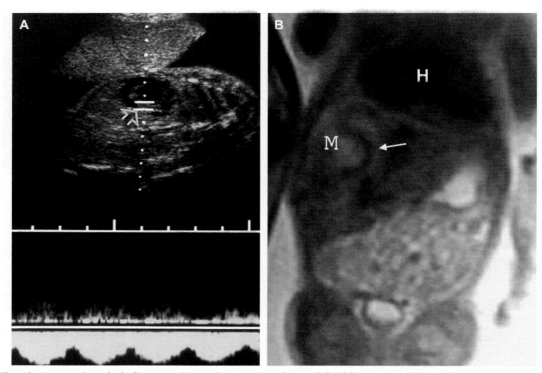

Fig. 12. Hemangioendothelioma at 28 weeks gestational age. (*A*) Oblique coronal Doppler sonogram shows a vascular mass in the liver. The Doppler gate is seen in the periphery of the mass. The tracing shows pulsatile venous flow. (*B*) Coronal T2-weighted image shows the vascular mass (*M*) in the liver. The liver is secondarily enlarged. A large draining vein is present with flow void (*arrow*). Because of the cardiac enlargement and concern for impending hydrops, the patient was treated with steroids and the lesion regressed in utero and resolved postnatally. (*Reproduced from* Morris J, Abbott J, Burrows P, et al. Antenatal diagnosis of fetal hepatic hemangioma treated with maternal corticosteroids. Obstet Gynecol 1999;94(5 Pt 2):813–5; with permission.)

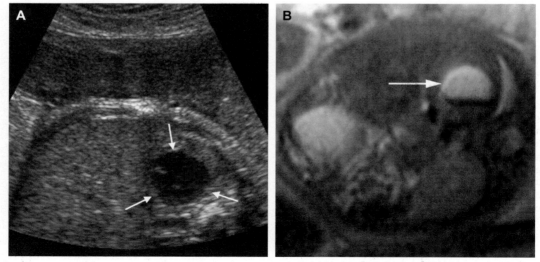

Fig. 13. Neuroblastoma at 33 weeks gestational age. (*A*) Transverse sonogram shows a complex cyst (*arrows*) in the right upper quadrant. (*B*) Axial T2-weighted image (oriented to maternal anatomy to best illustrate the fluid level) shows a fluid–fluid level within the cyst (*arrow*), suggesting layering hemorrhage. Histology showed a cystic neuroblastoma.

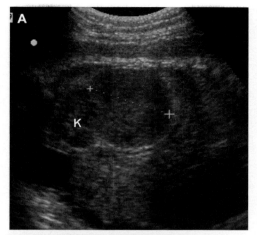

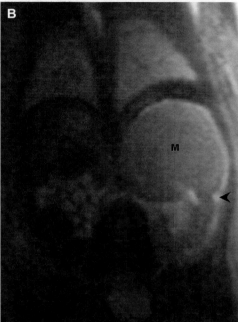

Fig. 14. Mesoblastic nephroma at 38 weeks gestational age. (*A*) Transverse sonogram shows a solid mass (*calipers*) above kidney (*K*). The adrenal gland was not visualized separately. (*B*) Coronal T2-weighted image depicts a well-circumscribed solid mass (*M*) arising from the upper pole of the kidney. A claw sign (*arrowhead*) demonstrates that this arises from the kidney. On other images (not shown) the adrenal gland was visualized separately from the mass. The most common solid renal neoplasm in utero is mesoblastic nephroma, which was found at histology (*B*). (*From* Levine D. Compendium of fetal MRI. Available at: bidmc.harvard.edu/content/bidmc/departments/radiology/files/fetalatlas/default.htm; with permission.)

are more commonly observed in the third trimester [106]. MR imaging may be helpful in distinguishing between sequestration and hemorrhagic adrenal lesions [113].

Renal tumors

Fetal renal tumors are rare. The most common solid renal neoplasm in utero is mesoblastic nephroma (Fig. 14). The sonographic finding is that of a solid homogeneous echogenic mass, indistinguishable from Wilms tumor [114,115]. There may be cystic areas caused by degeneration and hemorrhage [116] and high blood flow can be seen on Doppler evaluation [17]. MR imaging can be helpful in distinguishing between an upper pole renal mass and an adrenal lesion [78,117].

Polyhydramnios (likely secondary to polyuria) and hypercalcemia may occur [118]. The outcome from mesoblastic nephroma is excellent if complications do not occur in utero.

Pelvic and distal spine tumors

Sacrococcygeal teratoma (SCT, Fig. 15) is the most common tumor of the fetus and neonate, occurring in 1/40,000 live births. There is an association with neural tube defects, other spinal anomalies, and twins [119,120]. The main differential diagnosis of a cystic exophytic pelvic lesion is between the SCT and distal neural tube defect. Distal neural tube defects demonstrate splaying of the posterior element. In addition, with neural tube defects there is typically an associated Chiari malformation in the posterior fossa and elevated α-fetoprotein. Doppler examination does not demonstrate flow to the lesion.

SCT usually presents as a large midline exophytic mass posterior–inferior to the distal spine. The spine may demonstrate mass effect from the lesion, but there is not the splayed posterior elements seen in neural tube defect. SCT may be almost entirely external (type I), internal and external in equal parts (type II), mainly internal (type III), or entirely internal (type IV), according to the American Academy of Pediatrics Surgical Section (AAPSS) classification [121–123]. This classification system aids in counseling, operative planning, and possible fetal intervention [121–123]. Tumor size, vascularity, associated abnormalities, hemorrhage, hydrops, and polyhydramnios affect perinatal morbidity and mortality [3,122].

Because of high metabolic demand, vascular steal, and secondary high-output cardiac insufficiency, the prognosis for fetuses who have solid vascular tumors is usually grim [122]. Maternal discomfort from polyhydramnios, preterm labor, and rupture prevention can be treated with cyst aspiration and amnioreduction. Open fetal surgery is considered for debulking of SCT if there are signs of impending hydrops, gestational age less than 30 weeks, and favorable anatomy (AAPSS

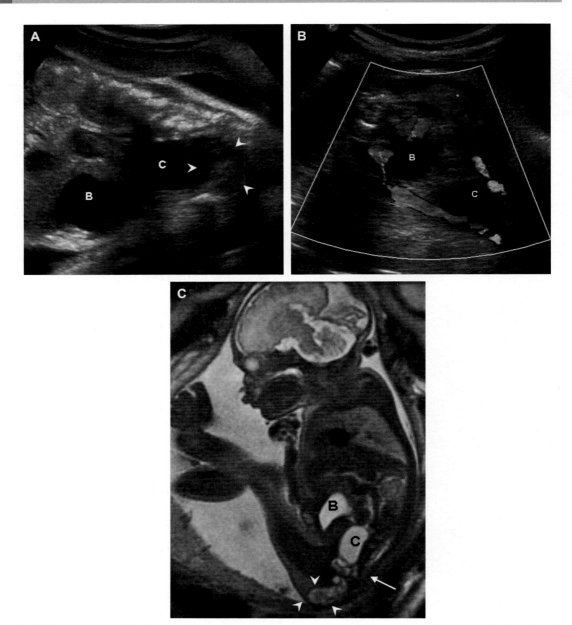

Fig. 15. Sacrococcygeal teratoma at 32 weeks gestational age. (*A*) Sagittal sonogram shows a cystic (*c*) and solid (*arrowheads*) mass anterior to the spine. The bladder is displaced superiorly. (*B*) Oblique coronal sonogram with color Doppler shows the umbilical arteries lateral to the bladder and the cystic part of the teratoma. (*C*) Sagittal T2-weighted image clearly delineates the extent of the sacrococcygeal teratoma. Because this is predominately intrapelvic with only a small extrapelvic extent, it is a grade III sacrococcygeal teratoma on the American Academy of Pediatrics Surgical Section (AAPSS) scale.

classification type I or II). A pre-eclamptic condition (mirror syndrome [124]), in which the mother's condition begins to mirror that of the sick fetus, is considered a contraindication to fetal intervention and should be treated with delivery [122,125,126].

MR imaging can aid in determining the precise location and extension of SCT [127–129]. If the SCT is entirely internal and cystic (15% of the cases), differentiation with anterior myelomeningocele and cloacal malformation should be considered [127,130].

Soft-tissue tumors of the extremities

A soft vascular tumor found in the extremity of the fetus is most likely to be a hemangioma. If cutaneous or subcutaneous cystic or multicystic lesions are seen in association with abnormal limb development (enlargement), this raises suspicion of Klippel-Trenaunay-Weber syndrome. Hemangiomas can grow rapidly with high-output cardiac failure, leading to fetal demise [131–133].

Infantile myofibromatosis (or hamartomatosis) has an incidence of 1 in 150,000 live births and is the most common nonvascular soft-tissue tumor. Echogenic masses on the back with calcifications are the main features [134].

Congenital fibrosarcoma is a malignant fibroblast tumor that usually involves the arm or leg. Unlike in adults, the process in the fetus usually has a lower malignant potential. Sonographic features are that of a homogeneous, echogenic, or mixed echogenicity soft-tissue tumor [135].

Summary

The diagnosis of a fetal neoplasm requires knowledge of how the location and appearance of the lesion affects the differential diagnosis. Gray-scale ultrasound, Doppler ultrasound, and MR imaging are tools that aid in making specific diagnosis and in predicting outcome, thus aiding patient counseling and preparation for delivery. Advances in fetal care, such as fetal surgery for sacrococcygeal teratomas with impending hydrops and EXIT procedure for lesions that threaten the airway, have markedly changed the manner in which fetal tumors are managed.

References

[1] Werb P, Scurry J, Ostor A, et al. Survey of congenital tumors in perinatal necropsies. Pathology 1992;24(4):247–53.

[2] Albert A, Cruz O, Montaner A, et al. [Congenital solid tumors. A thirteen-year review]. Cir Pediatr 2004;17(3):133–6 [In Spanish].

[3] Woodward PJ, Sohaey R, Kennedy A, et al. From the archives of the AFIP: a comprehensive review of fetal tumors with pathologic correlation. Radiographics 2005;25(1):215–42.

[4] Bouchard S, Johnson MP, Flake AW, et al. The EXIT procedure: experience and outcome in 31 cases. J Pediatr Surg 2002;37(3):418–26.

[5] Oi S, Kokunai T, Matsumoto S. Congenital brain tumors in Japan (ISPN Cooperative Study): specific clinical features in neonates. Childs Nerv Syst. 1990;6(2):86–91.

[6] Mehta V, Chapman A, McNeely PD, et al. Latency between symptom onset and diagnosis of pediatric brain tumors: an Eastern Canadian geographic study. Neurosurgery 2002;51(2): 365–72.

[7] Isaacs H Jr. I. Perinatal brain tumors: a review of 250 cases. Pediatr Neurol 2002;27(4):249–61.

[8] Isaacs H Jr. II. Perinatal brain tumors: a review of 250 cases. Pediatr Neurol 2002;27(5): 333–42.

[9] Kamitomo M, Sameshima H, Uetsuhara K, et al. Fetal glioblastoma: rapid growth during the third trimester. Fetal Diagn Ther 1998;13(6): 339–42.

[10] Isaacs H Jr. Congenital and neonatal malignant tumors. A 28-year experience at Children's Hospital of Los Angeles. Am J Pediatr Hematol Oncol 1987;9(2):121–9.

[11] Winters JL, Wilson D, Davis DG. Congenital glioblastoma multiforme: a report of three cases and a review of the literature. J Neurol Sci 2001; 188(1–2):13–9.

[12] Morof DF, Levine D, Stringer KF, et al. Congenital glioblastoma multiforme: prenatal diagnosis on the basis of sonography and magnetic resonance imaging. J Ultrasound Med 2001; 20(12):1369–75.

[13] Heckel S, Favre R, Gasser B, et al. Prenatal diagnosis of a congenital astrocytoma: a case report and literature review. Ultrasound Obstet Gynecol 1995;5(1):63–6.

[14] Geraghty AV, Knott PD, Hanna HM. Prenatal diagnosis of fetal glioblastoma multiforme. Prenat Diagn 1989;9(9):613–6.

[15] Guibaud L, Champion F, Buenerd A, et al. Fetal intraventricular glioblastoma: ultrasonographic, magnetic resonance imaging, and pathologic findings. J Ultrasound Med 1997;16(4):285–8.

[16] Lee DY, Kim YM, Yoo SJ, et al. Congenital glioblastoma diagnosed by fetal sonography. Childs Nerv Syst 1999;15(4):197–201.

[17] Chuang YM, Guo WY, Ho DM, et al. Skew ocular deviation: a catastrophic sign on MRI of fetal glioblastoma. Childs Nerv Syst 2003;19(5–6): 371–5.

[18] Buetow PC, Smirniotopoulos JG, Done S. Congenital brain tumors: a review of 45 cases. AJR Am J Roentgenol 1990;155(3):587–93.

[19] Sato T, Shimoda A, Takahashi T, et al. Congenital cerebellar neuroepithelial tumor with multiple divergent differentiations. Acta Neuropathol (Berl) 1980;50(2):143–6.

[20] Helmke K, Hausdorf G, Moehrs D, et al. CCT and sonographic findings in congenital craniopharyngioma. Neuroradiology 1984;26(6):523–6.

[21] Kultursay N, Gelal F, Mutluer S, et al. Antenatally diagnosed neonatal craniopharyngioma. J Perinatol 1995;15(5):426–8.

[22] Benli K, Cataltepe O, Oge HK, et al. Giant congenital meningioma in a newborn. Childs Nerv Syst 1990;6(8):462–4.

[23] van Vliet MA, Bravenboer B, Kock HC, et al. Congenital meningeal sarcoma—a case report. J Perinat Med 1983;11(5):249–54.

[24] Price DB, Miller LJ, Drexler S, et al. Congenital ganglioglioma: report of a case with an unusual imaging appearance. Pediatr Radiol 1997; 27(9):748–9.

[25] Comi AM, Backstrom JW, Burger PC, et al. Clinical and neuroradiologic findings in infants with intracranial ependymomas. Pediatric Oncology Group. Pediatr Neurol 1998;18(1):23–9.

[26] Kudo H, Oi S, Tamaki N, et al. Ependymoma diagnosed in the first year of life in Japan in collaboration with the International Society for Pediatric Neurosurgery. Childs Nerv Syst 1990;6(7):375–8.

[27] Mitra AG, Dickerson C. Central nervous system tumor with associated unilateral ventriculomegaly: unusual prenatal presentation of subsequently diagnosed tuberous sclerosis. J Ultrasound Med 2000;19(9):651–4.

[28] Durfee SM, Kim FM, Benson CB. Postnatal outcome of fetuses with the prenatal diagnosis of asymmetric hydrocephalus. J Ultrasound Med 2001;20(3):263–8.

[29] Levine D, Barnes P, Korf B, et al. Tuberous sclerosis in the fetus: second-trimester diagnosis of subependymal tubers with ultrafast MR imaging. AJR Am J Roentgenol 2000;175(4):1067–9.

[30] Sonigo P. [Contribution of MRI in the evaluation of fetal malformations]. J Gynecol Obstet Biol Reprod 2000;29(3):269–71 [In French].

[31] Levine D, Barne P. MR of fetal CNS anomalies. In: Levine D, editor. Atlas of fetal MRI. 1st edition. Boca Raton (FL): Taylor & Francis Group; 2005.

[32] Lau TK, Leung TN, Leung TY, et al. Fetal scalp cysts: challenge in diagnosis and counseling. J Ultrasound Med 2001;20(2):175–7.

[33] Ogle RF, Jauniaux E. Fetal scalp cysts—dilemmas in diagnosis. Prenat Diagn 1999; 19(12):1157–9.

[34] Sabbagha RE, Tamura RK, Dal Compo S, et al. Fetal cranial and craniocervical masses: ultrasound characteristics and differential diagnosis. Am J Obstet Gynecol. 1980;138(5):511–7.

[35] Levine D. Compendium of fetal MRI. Available at: bidmc.harvard.edu/content/bidmc/departments/radiology/files/fetalatlas/default.htm. Boston; 2004.

[36] Treadwell MC, Sepulveda W, LeBlanc LL, et al. Prenatal diagnosis of fetal cutaneous hemangioma: case report and review of the literature. J Ultrasound Med 1993;12(11):683–7.

[37] Boon LM, Enjolras O, Mulliken JB. Congenital hemangioma: evidence of accelerated involution. J Pediatr 1996;128(3):329–35.

[38] Goncalves LF, Pereira ET, Parente LM, et al. Cutaneous hemangioma of the thigh: prenatal diagnosis. Ultrasound Obstet Gynecol 1997; 9(2):128–30.

[39] Winter TC 3rd, Mack LA, Cyr DR. Prenatal sonographic diagnosis of scalp edema/cephalohematoma mimicking an encephalocele. AJR Am J Roentgenol 1993;161(6):1247–8.

[40] Pascual-Castroviejo I. The association of extracranial and intracranial vascular malformations in children. Can J Neurol Sci 1985;12(2): 139–48.

[41] Mitchell CS. Vertex hemangioma mimicking an encephalocele. J Am Osteopath Assoc 1999; 99(12):626–7.

[42] Shipp TD, Bromley B, Benacerraf B. The ultrasonographic appearance and outcome for fetuses with masses distorting the fetal face. J Ultrasound Med 1995;14(9):673–8.

[43] Hubbard AM, Crombleholme TM, Adzick NS. Prenatal MRI evaluation of giant neck masses in preparation for the fetal exit procedure. Am J Perinatol 1998;15(4):253–7.

[44] Liechty KW, Crombleholme TM, Flake AW, et al. Intrapartum airway management for giant fetal neck masses: the EXIT (ex utero intrapartum treatment) procedure. Am J Obstet Gynecol 1997;177(4):870–4.

[45] Witters I, Moerman P, Louwagie D, et al. Second trimester prenatal diagnosis of epignathus teratoma in ring X chromosome mosaicism with inactive ring X chromosome. Ann Genet 2001;44(4):179–82.

[46] Pavlin JE, O'Gorman A, Williams HB, et al. Epignathus: a report of two cases. Ann Plast Surg 1984;13(5):452–6.

[47] Isaacs H Jr. Perinatal (fetal and neonatal) germ cell tumors. J Pediatr Surg 2004;39(7):1003–13.

[48] Clement K, Chamberlain P, Boyd P, et al. Prenatal diagnosis of an epignathus: a case report and review of the literature. Ultrasound Obstet Gynecol 2001;18(2):178–81.

[49] Morof D, Levine D, Grable I, et al. Oropharyngeal teratoma: prenatal diagnosis and assessment using sonography, MRI, and CT with management by ex utero intrapartum treatment procedure. AJR Am J Roentgenol 2004;183(2): 493–6.

[50] Garmel SH, Crombleholme TM, Semple JP, et al. Prenatal diagnosis and management of fetal tumors. Semin Perinatol 1994;18(4): 350–65.

[51] Respondek-Liberska M, Janiak K, Jakubek A, et al. Prenatal diagnosis of fetal face hemangioma in a case of Kasabach-Merritt syndrome. Ultrasound Obstet Gynecol 2002;19(6):627–9.

[52] Isaacs Hart J. Germ cell tumors. In: Isaacs Hart J, editor. Tumors of the fetus and newborn. Philadelphia: Saunders; 1997. p. 1–38.

[53] O'Callaghan MG, House M, Ebay S, et al. Rhabdomyoma of the head and neck demonstrated by prenatal magnetic resonance imaging. J Comput Assist Tomogr. 2005;29(1):130–2.

[54] Carron JD, Darrow DH, Karakla DW. Fetal rhabdomyoma of the posterior cervical triangle. Int J Pediatr Otorhinolaryngol 2001;61(1): 77–81.

[55] Roy S, Sinsky A, Williams B, et al. Congenital epulis: prenatal imaging with MRI and ultrasound. Pediatr Radiol 2003;33(11):800–3.

[56] Maat-Kievit JA, Oepkes D, Hartwig NG, et al. A large retinoblastoma detected in a fetus at 21 weeks of gestation. Prenat Diagn 1993; 13(5):377–84.

[57] Levine D, Stroustrup Smith A. MR imaging of the fetal skull, face, and neck. In: Levine D, editor. Atlas of Fetal MRI. Boca Raton, FL: Taylor & Francis; 2005. p. 73–90.

[58] van Oppen AC, Breslau-Siderius EJ, Stoutenbeek P, et al. A fetal cystic neck mass associated with maternal tuberous sclerosis. Case report and literature review. Prenat Diagn 1991;11(12):915–20.

[59] Thomas RL. Prenatal diagnosis of giant cystic hygroma: prognosis, counselling, and management; case presentation and review of the recent literature. Prenat Diagn 1992;12(11): 919–23.

[60] Axt-Fliedner R, Hendrik HJ, Schwaiger C, et al. Prenatal and perinatal aspects of a giant fetal cervicothoracal lymphangioma. Fetal Diagn Ther 2002;17(1):3–7.

[61] Deshpande P, Twining P, O'Neill D. Prenatal diagnosis of fetal abdominal lymphangioma by ultrasonography. Ultrasound Obstet Gynecol 2001;17(5):445–8.

[62] Senoh D, Hanaoka U, Tanaka Y, et al. Antenatal ultrasonographic features of fetal giant hemangiolymphangioma. Ultrasound Obstet Gynecol 2001;17(3):252–4.

[63] Tanriverdi HA, Ertan AK, Hendrik HJ, et al. Outcome of cystic hygroma in fetuses with normal karyotypes depends on associated findings. Eur J Obstet Gynecol Reprod Biol 2005;118(1): 40–6.

[64] Bronshtein M, Bar-Hava I, Blumenfeld I, et al. The difference between septated and nonseptated nuchal cystic hygroma in the early second trimester. Obstet Gynecol 1993;81(5 (Pt 1)): 683–7.

[65] Brumfield CG, Wenstrom KD, Davis RO, et al. Second-trimester cystic hygroma: prognosis of septated and nonseptated lesions. Obstet Gynecol 1996;88(6):979–82.

[66] Lee SH, Cho JY, Song MJ, et al. Prenatal ultrasound findings of fetal neoplasms. Korean J Radiol 2002;3(1):64–73.

[67] Kaminopetros P, Jauniaux E, Kane P, et al. Prenatal diagnosis of an extensive fetal lymphangioma using ultrasonography, magnetic resonance imaging and cytology. Br J Radiol 1997;70(835):750–3.

[68] Machado LE, Osborne NG, Bonilla-Musoles F. Three-dimensional sonographic diagnosis of a large cystic neck lymphangioma. J Ultrasound Med 2004;23(6):877–81.

[69] Shiraishi H, Nakamura M, Ichihashi K, et al. Prenatal MRI in a fetus with a giant neck hemangioma: a case report. Prenat Diagn 2000; 20(12):1004–7.

[70] Morine M, Takeda T, Minekawa R, et al. Antenatal diagnosis and treatment of a case of fetal goitrous hypothyroidism associated with high-output cardiac failure. Ultrasound Obstet Gynecol 2002;19(5):506–9.

[71] Abuhamad AZ, Fisher DA, Warsof SL, et al. Antenatal diagnosis and treatment of fetal goitrous hypothyroidism: case report and review of the literature. Ultrasound Obstet Gynecol 1995; 6(5):368–71.

[72] Gruner C, Kollert A, Wildt L, et al. Intrauterine treatment of fetal goitrous hypothyroidism controlled by determination of thyroid-stimulating hormone in fetal serum. A case report and review of the literature. Fetal Diagn Ther 2001; 16(1):47–51.

[73] Levine D. MR imaging of fetal thoracic abnormalities. In: Levine D, editor. Atlas of Fetal MRI. Boca Raton: Taylor & Francis Group; 2005. p. 91–112.

[74] Hayashi A, Kikuchi A, Matsumoto Y, et al. Massive cystic lymphangiomas of a fetus. Congenit Anom (Kyoto) 2005;45(4):154–6.

[75] Kozlowski KJ, Frazier CN, Quirk JG Jr. Prenatal diagnosis of abdominal cystic hygroma. Prenat Diagn 1988;8(6):405–9.

[76] Liang RI, Wang P, Chang FM, et al. Prenatal sonographic characteristics and Doppler blood flow study in a case of a large fetal mediastinal teratoma. Ultrasound Obstet Gynecol 1998; 11(3):214–8.

[77] Froberg MK, Brown RE, Maylock J, et al. In utero development of a mediastinal teratoma: a second-trimester event. Prenat Diagn 1994; 14(9):884–7.

[78] Williams G, Coakley FV, Qayyum A, et al. Fetal relative lung volume: quantification by using prenatal MR imaging lung volumetry. Radiology 2004;233(2):457–62.

[79] Bader R, Hornberger LK, Nijmeh LJ, et al. Fetal pericardial teratoma: presentation of two cases and review of literature. Am J Perinatol 2006; 23(1):53–8.

[80] Sklansky M, Greenberg M, Lucas V, et al. Intrapericardial teratoma in a twin fetus: diagnosis and management. Obstet Gynecol 1997;89(5 Pt 2): 807–9.

[81] Tollens M, Grab D, Lang D, et al. Pericardial teratoma: prenatal diagnosis and course. Fetal Diagn Ther 2003;18(6):432–6.

[82] Wallace G, Smith HC, Watson GH, et al. Tuberous sclerosis presenting with fetal and neonatal cardiac tumours. Arch Dis Child 1990; 65(4 Spec No):377–9.

[83] Krapp M, Baschat AA, Gembruch U, et al. Tuberous sclerosis with intracardiac rhabdomyoma in a fetus with trisomy 21: case report and review of literature. Prenat Diagn 1999; 19(7):610–3.

[84] Wei J, Li P, Chiriboga L, et al. Tuberous sclerosis in a 19-week fetus: immunohistochemical and molecular study of hamartin and tuberin. Pediatr Dev Pathol 2002;5(5): 448–64.

[85] King JA, Stamilio DM. Maternal and fetal tuberous sclerosis complicating pregnancy: a case report and overview of the literature. Am J Perinatol 2005;22(2):103–8.

[86] D'Addario V, Selvaggio S, Pinto V, et al. Fetal subependymal cysts with normal neonatal outcome. A case report. Fetal Diagn Ther 2003; 18(3):170–3.

[87] Pipitone S, Mongiovi M, Grillo R, et al. Cardiac rhabdomyoma in intrauterine life: clinical features and natural history. A case series and review of published reports. Ital Heart J 2002; 3(1):48–52.

[88] Chou SY, Chiang HK, Chow PK, et al. Fetal hepatic hemangioma diagnosed prenatally with ultrasonography. Acta Obstet Gynecol Scand 2005;84(3):301–2.

[89] Gembruch U, Baschat AA, Gloeckner-Hoffmann K, et al. Prenatal diagnosis and management of fetuses with liver hemangiomata. Ultrasound Obstet Gynecol 2002;19(5): 454–60.

[90] Abuhamad AZ, Lewis D, Inati MN, et al. The use of color flow Doppler in the diagnosis of fetal hepatic hemangioma. J Ultrasound Med 1993;12(4):223–6.

[91] Chuileannain FN, Rowlands S, Sampson A. Ultrasonographic appearances of fetal hepatic hemangioma. J Ultrasound Med 1999;18(5): 379–81.

[92] Sepulveda WH, Donetch G, Giuliano A. Prenatal sonographic diagnosis of fetal hepatic hemangioma. Eur J Obstet Gynecol Reprod Biol 1993;48(1):73–6.

[93] Wu TJ, Teng RJ. Diffuse neonatal haemangiomatosis with intra-uterine haemorrhage and hydrops fetalis: a case report. Eur J Pediatr 1994;153(10):759–61.

[94] Gonen R, Fong K, Chiasson DA. Prenatal sonographic diagnosis of hepatic hemangioendothelioma with secondary nonimmune hydrops fetalis. Obstet Gynecol 1989;73(3 Pt 2):485–7.

[95] Dachman AH, Lichtenstein JE, Friedman AC, et al. Infantile hemangioendothelioma of the liver: a radiologic-pathologic-clinical correlation. AJR Am J Roentgenol 1983;140(6):1091–6.

[96] Boulot P, Deschamps F, Montoya F, et al. Prenatal aspects of giant fetal cranial haemangioendothelioma. Prenat Diagn 1996;16(4): 357–9.

[97] Kush ML, Weiner CP, Harman CR, et al. Lethal progression of a fetal intracranial arteriovenous malformation. J Ultrasound Med 2003;22(6): 645–8.

[98] Morimura Y, Fujimori K, Ishida T, et al. Fetal hepatic hemangioma representing non-reassuring pattern in fetal heart rate monitoring. J Obstet Gynaecol Res 2003;29(5):347–50.

[99] Weber TR, Connors RH, Tracy TF Jr, et al. Complex hemangiomas of infants and children. Individualized management in 22 cases. Arch Surg 1990;125(8):1017–20 [discussion: 1020–11].

[100] Morris J, Abbott J, Burrows P, et al. Antenatal diagnosis of fetal hepatic hemangioma treated with maternal corticosteroids. Obstet Gynecol 1999;94(5 Pt 2):813–5.

[101] Kamata S, Nose K, Sawai T, et al. Fetal mesenchymal hamartoma of the liver: report of a case. J Pediatr Surg 2003;38(4):639–41.

[102] Marks F, Thomas P, Lustig I, et al. In utero sonographic description of a fetal liver adenoma. J Ultrasound Med 1990;9(2):119–22.

[103] Applegate KE, Ghei M, Perez-Atayde AR. Prenatal detection of a solitary liver adenoma. Pediatr Radiol 1999;29(2):92–4.

[104] Toma P, Lucigrai G, Marzoli A, et al. Prenatal diagnosis of metastatic adrenal neuroblastoma with sonography and MR imaging. AJR Am J Roentgenol 1994;162(5):1183–4.

[105] Aviram R, Cohen IJ, Kornreich L, et al. Prenatal imaging of fetal hepatoblastoma. J Matern Fetal Neonatal Med 2005;17(2):157–9.

[106] Curtis MR, Mooney DP, Vaccaro TJ, et al. Prenatal ultrasound characterization of the suprarenal mass: distinction between neuroblastoma and subdiaphragmatic extralobar pulmonary sequestration. J Ultrasound Med 1997;16(2):75–83.

[107] Gocmen R, Basaran C, Karcaaltincaba M, et al. Bilateral hemorrhagic adrenal cysts in an incomplete form of Beckwith-Wiedemann syndrome: MRI and prenatal US findings. Abdom Imaging 2005;30(6):786–9.

[108] Deeg KH, Bettendorf U, Hofmann V. Differential diagnosis of neonatal adrenal haemorrhage and congenital neuroblastoma by colour coded Doppler sonography and power Doppler sonography. Eur J Pediatr 1998; 157(4):294–7.

[109] Jaffa AJ, Many A, Hartoov J, et al. Prenatal sonographic diagnosis of metastatic neuroblastoma: report of a case and review of the literature. Prenat Diagn 1993;13(1):73–7.

[110] Gorincour G, Dugougeat-Pilleul F, Bouvier R, et al. Prenatal presentation of cervical congenital neuroblastoma. Prenat Diagn 2003;23(8):690–3.

[111] Yamagiwa I, Obata K, Saito H. Prenatally detected cystic neuroblastoma. Pediatr Surg Int 1998;13(2–3):215–7.

[112] Lee W, Comstock CH, Jurcak-Zaleski S. Prenatal diagnosis of adrenal hemorrhage by ultrasonography. J Ultrasound Med 1992;11(7):369–71.

[113] Sauvat F, Sarnacki S, Brisse H, et al. Outcome of suprarenal localized masses diagnosed during the perinatal period: a retrospective multicenter study. Cancer 2002;94(9):2474–80.

[114] Applegate KE, Ghei M, Perez-Atayde AR. Prenatal detection of a Wilms' tumor. Pediatr Radiol 1999;29(1):65–7.

[115] Apuzzio JJ, Unwin W, Adhate A, et al. Prenatal diagnosis of fetal renal mesoblastic nephroma. Am J Obstet Gynecol 1986;154(3):636–7.

[116] Murthi GV, Carachi R, Howatson A. Congenital cystic mesoblastic nephroma. Pediatr Surg Int 2003;19(1–2):109–11.

[117] Chen WY, Lin CN, Chao CS, et al. Prenatal diagnosis of congenital mesoblastic nephroma in mid-second trimester by sonography and magnetic resonance imaging. Prenat Diagn 2003;23(11):927–31.

[118] Fung TY, Fung YM, Ng PC, et al. Polyhydramnios and hypercalcemia associated with congenital mesoblastic nephroma: case report and a new appraisal. Obstet Gynecol 1995;85(5 Pt 2):815–7.

[119] Flake AW, Harrison MR, Adzick NS, et al. Fetal sacrococcygeal teratoma. J Pediatr Surg 1986; 21(7):563–6.

[120] Coleman BG, Adzick NS, Crombleholme TM, et al. Fetal therapy: state of the art. J Ultrasound Med 2002;21(11):1257–88.

[121] Altman RP, Randolph JG, Lilly JR. Sacrococcygeal teratoma: American Academy of Pediatrics Surgical Section Survey–1973. J Pediatr Surg 1974;9(3):389–98.

[122] Hedrick HL, Flake AW, Crombleholme TM, et al. Sacrococcygeal teratoma: prenatal assessment, fetal intervention, and outcome. J Pediatr Surg 2004;39(3):430–8.

[123] Kirkinen P, Partanen K, Merikanto J, et al. Ultrasonic and magnetic resonance imaging of fetal sacrococcygeal teratoma. Acta Obstet Gynecol Scand 1997;76(10):917–22.

[124] Bond SJ, Harrison MR, Schmidt KG, et al. Death due to high-output cardiac failure in fetal sacrococcygeal teratoma. J Pediatr Surg 1990;25(12):1287–91.

[125] Alter DN, Reed KL, Marx GR, et al. Prenatal diagnosis of congestive heart failure in a fetus with a sacrococcygeal teratoma. Obstet Gynecol 1988;71(6 Pt 2):978–81.

[126] Adzick NS, Crombleholme TM, Morgan MA, et al. A rapidly growing fetal teratoma. Lancet 1997;349(9051):538.

[127] Chen CP, Sheu JC, Huang JK, et al. Second-trimester magnetic resonance imaging of fetal sacrococcygeal teratoma with intrapelvic extension in a co-twin. Prenat Diagn 2004; 24(12):1015–7.

[128] Garel C, Mizouni L, Menez F, et al. Prenatal diagnosis of a cystic type IV sacrococcygeal teratoma mimicking a cloacal anomaly: contribution of MR. Prenat Diagn 2005;25(3): 216–9.

[129] Veyrac C, Couture A, Saguintaah M, et al. MRI of fetal GI tract abnormalities. Abdom Imaging 2004;29(4):411–20.

[130] Wakhlu A, Misra S, Tandon RK, et al. Sacrococcygeal teratoma. Pediatr Surg Int 2002;18(5–6): 384–7.

[131] Roberts RV, Dickinson JE, Hugo PJ, et al. Prenatal sonographic appearances of Klippel-Trenaunay-Weber syndrome. Prenat Diagn 1999; 19(4):369–71.

[132] Goncalves LF, Rojas MV, Vitorello D, et al. Klippel-Trenaunay-Weber syndrome presenting as massive lymphangiohemangioma of the thigh: prenatal diagnosis. Ultrasound Obstet Gynecol 2000;15(6):537–41.

[133] Paladini D, Lamberti A, Teodoro A, et al. Prenatal diagnosis and hemodynamic evaluation of Klippel-Trenaunay-Weber syndrome. Ultrasound Obstet Gynecol 1998;12(3):215–7.

[134] Meizner I, Shalev J, Mashiach R, et al. Prenatal ultrasound diagnosis of infantile myofibromatosis—a case report. Ultrasound Obstet Gynecol 2000;16(1):84–6.

[135] Tseng JJ, Chou MM, Li MC, et al. Prenatal sonographic appearance of congenital axillary fibrosarcoma with intrathoracic invasion. Ultrasound Obstet Gynecol 2002;20(1): 98–100.

ELSEVIER
SAUNDERS

ULTRASOUND
CLINICS

Ultrasound Clin 2 (2007) 265

Preface

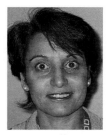

Sheila Sheth, MD
Department of Radiology
Johns Hopkins University
600 North Wolfe Street
Baltimore, MD 21287, USA

E-mail address:
ssheth@jhmi.edu

Sheila Sheth, MD
Guest Editor

Ultrasound remains the imaging modality of choice in the evaluation of suspected gynecologic pathology. Increasingly, however, magnetic resonance and CT are being performed for this indication. In the best of cases, CT—and particularly MR—are being requested as a problem-solving modality, for accurate location of pelvic masses or for staging of gynecologic malignancies, and provide invaluable additional information. On the other hand, in the patient with acute pelvic or lower abdominal pain, CT is too often the first imaging test ordered by the emergency department physician because it is readily available, fast, and not operator dependent, exposing young women to unnecessary radiation. In any case, the sonologist needs to become familiar with the appropriate indications and the appearances of a variety of gynecologic diseases on these modalities.

In this issue of *Ultrasound Clinics*, the editors have gathered a group of articles emphasizing correlative imaging between ultrasound, CT, and MR, discussing appropriate indications for each of these modalities.

The article by Drs. Sheth and Macura discusses the respective role of ultrasound and MR in diseases affecting the uterine myometrium, emphasizing the invaluable contribution of MR for the planning of uterine myoma embolization, as well as the diagnosis of adenomyosis. The article by Drs. Horrow, Rodgers, and Naqvi reviews the findings of acute and chronic pelvic inflammatory disease and discusses the advantages offered by CT in complex cases, as well as techniques to optimize the CT exam. The article by Drs. Scoutt, Balarowich, and Lev-Toaff presents the imaging findings associated with ovarian torsion.

doi:10.1016/j.cult.2007.11.002

ULTRASOUND
CLINICS

Ultrasound Clin 2 (2007) 267–295

Sonography of the Uterine Myometrium: Myomas and Beyond

Sheila Sheth, MD*, Katarzyna Macura, MD

Suspected abnormality of the uterine myometrium is one of the most common indications for pelvic sonography. Uterine myomas are among the most frequently encountered pelvic masses, affecting up to 20% to 50% of women. Adenomyosis is another common condition that was often overlooked on imaging until a few years ago. Up until recently, hysterectomy was the treatment of choice for women who had symptomatic myomas, intractable vaginal bleeding, or dysmenorrhea, who did not desire further pregnancy.

As more women are interested in newer, less-invasive therapeutic options, refinement of imaging techniques and diagnoses becomes critical to select optimal management.

This article reviews the sonographic appearance of myomas with emphasis on those findings that are important for management and discusses the sonographic diagnosis of adenomyosis. This review is followed by a brief discussion of less common pathologic conditions affecting the myometrium, such as sarcomas and arteriovenous malformations.

Department of Radiology, School of Medicine, Johns Hopkins University, 600 North Wolfe Street, Baltimore, MD 21287, USA
* Corresponding author.
E-mail address: ssheth@jhmi.edu (S. Sheth).

1556-858X/07/$ – see front matter © 2007 Elsevier Inc. All rights reserved.
ultrasound.theclinics.com

doi:10.1016/j.cult.2007.08.011

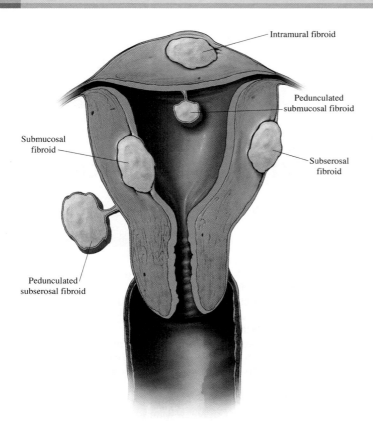

Intramural fibroid

Pedunculated
submucosal fibroid

Submucosal
fibroid

Subserosal
fibroid

Pedunculated
subserosal fibroid

Fig. 1. Various locations of myomas. (*Courtesy of* Frank M. Corl, MS, Baltimore, MD.)

Finally, the role of pelvic MR imaging as a problem-solving modality for evaluation of the myometrium is addressed.

Uterine myomas

Myomas, also called leiomyomas or fibroids, are benign tumors arising from the smooth muscle of the uterus. In addition to smooth muscle, most myomas contain varying amount of fibrous tissue. They are most commonly seen in the fourth and fifth decades and their growth is estrogen-dependent [1]. Myomas are three to nine times more common in black women, tend to be larger than in the white population, and are more frequently symptomatic at a younger age [2].

Although myomas are found in up to 77% of hysterectomy specimens and are often multiple [3], they become symptomatic in approximately 25% of patients. Common symptoms include menorrhagia, sometimes severe enough to result in iron-deficiency anemia; pelvic pain or pressure; and infertility [4]. The location of a myoma is an important factor determining symptoms. Most myomas are intramural and may produce mass effect on surrounding structures when they reach a large size. Although only 10% to 15% of myomas are

submucosal, they are usually symptomatic because distortion of the endometrial cavity leads to bleeding, infertility, or recurrent abortion. If the growth of the myoma is predominantly toward the periphery of the uterus, it is classified as subserosal. Occasionally, these subserosal myomas may become pedunculated and even outgrow their uterine blood supply and become parasitic (Fig. 1).

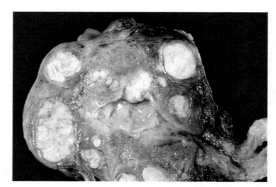

Fig. 2. Gross pathologic specimen of a uterine myoma. Multiple myomas are present. Note the pseudocapsule.

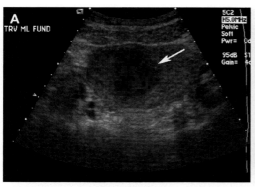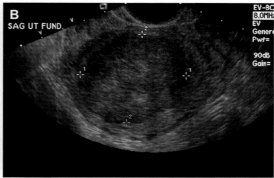

Fig. 3. A 36-year-old woman who has a history of infertility and irregular bleeding. (*A*) Transabdominal sonography of the uterus, transverse image, shows a hypoechoic mass in the uterine fundus (*arrow*). (*B*) Endovaginal sonography of the uterus, sagittal image, better depicts a hypoechoic mass with well-defined borders (between calipers). The presence of a single myoma was confirmed by myomectomy.

Treatment options for symptomatic myomas

Hysterectomy is the traditional treatment of symptomatic myomas and remains one of the most common surgical procedures performed in the United States. As the title of a recent *New England Journal of Medicine*, "Treatment of Uterine Fibroids—Is Surgery Obsolete?" indicates [5], several new less radical and less invasive treatment options are now available to women who desire future pregnancies or opt to keep their uterus for other reasons. In addition to uterine-preserving surgical techniques, such as abdominal or hysteroscopic myomectomies, new therapies include uterine artery embolization (UAE), MR-guided focused ultrasound, and medical management with gonadotropin-releasing hormone (GnRH) agonists. Many of these new techniques require more sophisticated imaging techniques allowing a definitive diagnosis of myomas and precise mapping of their number and location.

Sonographic diagnosis of myomas

Sonography remains the most frequently performed and cost-effective imaging modality to evaluate patients who have suspected myomas. Compared with transabdominal sonography (TAS), endovaginal sonography (EVS) allows better detection of small myomas and diagnosis of submucosal location. Because of the lower penetration and limited field of view of the vaginal transducers, however, EVS can have considerable limitations in patients who have large tumors. In our laboratory, TAS with 2- to 4-MHz sector or curvilinear transducer always precedes EVS, at least for the initial examination. Because large pelvic masses, if present, would displace small bowel loops and be readily visualized, we do not require patients to have a full bladder.

Sonographic appearance

The sonographic appearance of myomas is well documented [6]. The uterus may be enlarged with a smooth or lobulated contour. Because the surrounding myometrium is compressed and forms a pseudocapsule, myomas have well-defined borders (Fig. 2). Small tumors are typically relatively hypoechoic compared with the surrounding myometrium, with poor sound transmission (Fig. 3). As they outgrow their relatively poor blood supply, at least two thirds of myoma undergo some form of degeneration, accounting for their variable echotexture (Fig. 4). Hyaline, cystic, myxoid, and red degeneration have been described. Some lesions have a relatively homogeneous echotexture, whereas others contain echogenic or cystic area (Fig. 5). Calcifications, either peripheral or punctuate, are not

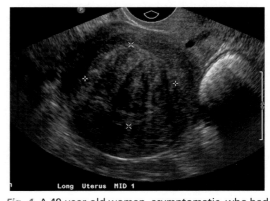

Fig. 4. A 49-year-old woman, asymptomatic, who had mildly enlarged uterus on pelvic examination. Endovaginal sonography of the uterus, sagittal image, shows a well-defined mildly heterogeneous mass in the myometrium (between calipers), an appearance characteristic of uterine myoma.

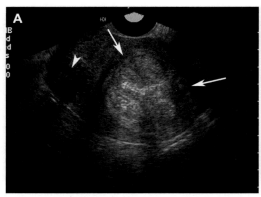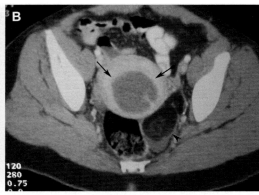

Fig. 5. A 42-year-old woman who had a 5-day history of pelvic pain. (*A*) Endovaginal sonography of the uterus, sagittal image, shows a well-defined echogenic mass in the myometrium (*arrows*). Note the smaller hypoechoic mass (*arrowhead*). (*B*) Contrast-enhanced axial CT of the pelvis shows a low attenuation intrauterine mass with rim enhancement suggestive of degenerating myoma (*arrows*). The left ovarian teratoma (*arrowhead*) was also seen on the pelvic ultrasound. The diagnosis of infarcted myoma was confirmed on the hysterectomy specimen.

rare (Figs. 6 and 7) [6]. A distinctive pattern of recurrent shadowing not originating from an echogenic focus is believed to be characteristic and allows specific diagnosis of myomas even if they are located in unusual locations (Fig. 8). Correlation with histologic specimen has shown that these shadows are produced by the refraction of the sound beam as it encounters interfaces between whorls of smooth muscles and fibrous connective tissue bands [7].

Sonographic evaluation of location

Intramural myomas

Intramural myoma is the most common location (see Figs. 3 and 4). Women who have intramural myomas are the best candidates for UAE.

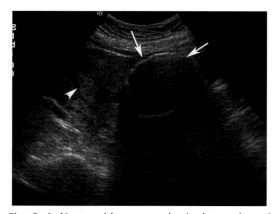

Fig. 6. A 41-year-old woman who had an enlarged uterus on physical examination. Transabdominal sonography of the uterus, sagittal image, shows a mass in the anterior myometrium with peripheral rim of calcifications (*arrows*). Arrowhead indicates endometrial stripe.

Submucosal myomas

Submucosal myomas distort the endometrial cavity and thus are often symptomatic. Patients may present with menorrhagia, recurrent pregnancy loss, or even infertility. Disruption and distortion of the endometrial stripe caused by submucosal myomas is best appreciated on EVS, unless the uterus is massively enlarged (Fig. 9). Purely intracavitary lesions are rare. When considering surgical management, it is critical to determine the proportion of the myoma that is projecting within the endometrial cavity: if more than 50% of the mass extends into the cavity, hysteroscopic removal is favored [8]. In equivocal cases, sonohysterography has been shown to provide additional information and improve diagnostic confidence (Fig. 10) [4].

Subserosal myomas

These lesions deform the contour of the uterus (Fig. 11). Pedunculated subserosal myomas become symptomatic if they cause pressure on adjacent organs. They present as exophytic solid masses with varying degree of attachment to the body of the uterus. Pedunculated myomas in the broad ligament may mimic a solid adnexal mass. The characteristic recurrent shadowing pattern associated with myomas is helpful in the differential diagnosis, although ovarian fibromas have similar acoustic characteristics. Another clue to the diagnosis of a pedunculated myoma is the visualization, on color Doppler, of blood vessels extending from the uterine body to the mass (Fig. 12). The presence of a separate ipsilateral ovary is also helpful in excluding a solid ovarian mass. Careful scanning with TAS, including examination of the adnexa and the pelvis above the uterine fundus, is critical to avoid missing very exophytic myomas.

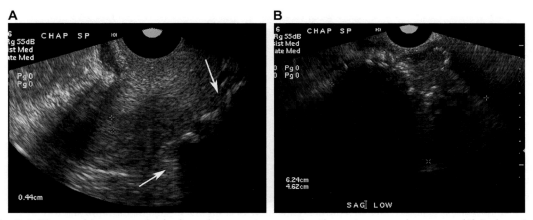

Fig. 7. A 73-year-old woman who had a pelvic mass compressing the rectum on colonoscopy. (*A*) Endovaginal sonography of the uterus, sagittal image, shows a small postmenopausal uterus. Note area of shadowing posterior to the uterus (*arrows*). (*B*) Endovaginal sonography, sagittal image, of this area shows a calcified mass (between calipers).

Cervical myomas

Cervical myomas are present in less than 1% of hysterectomy specimens [9] but they are an important potential cause of dystocia during labor. In nonpregnant women they are usually asymptomatic, unless they cause pressure symptoms on the bladder, urethra, or rectum [10].

Prolapsing myoma

Occasionally, a pedunculated fibroid submucosal myoma can prolapse through the cervix and present as a vaginal or cervical mass, usually in a woman seeking medical attention because of profuse vaginal bleeding (Fig. 13).

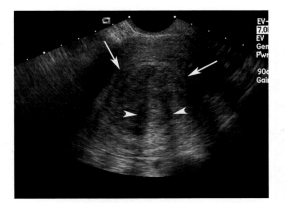

Fig. 8. A 49-year-old woman who had a history of myomas. Endovaginal sonography of the uterus, sagittal image, shows a well-defined mass in the uterus (*arrows*). Note areas of shadowing within the mass (*arrowheads*).

Role of imaging in the pre- and postprocedure evaluation of uterine artery embolization

Since it was first described in 1995 UAE for symptomatic uterine myomas has gained wide acceptance [11]. Preprocedure imaging is essential for appropriate patient selection, because the most important deciding factors include the size and location of the tumors [12]. UAE is most beneficial for intramural myomas. Purely submucosal lesions are best removed surgically. Pedunculated myomas with limited attachment to the uterine body should not be treated with UAE because of the risk for stalk infarction and subsequent detachment of the mass from the uterus and peritoneal irritation [12]. Calcified or necrotic myomas with poor vascular supply also respond less than optimally to embolization [13].

In the United States, women considering UAE often undergo pelvic MR for preprocedure planning to overcome some of the limitations of sonography. These limitations include inaccurate measurement of the size of myomas, particularly if the tumors are larger than the field of view of the transducer. In these cases, TAS is superior to EVS because of the latter limited field of view and penetration. It is also worthwhile to attempt TAS with extended field of view for better depiction of the myomas and their relationship with the uterus (Fig. 14). Other pitfalls include failure to identify pedunculated myomas and misdiagnosis of the exact location of myomas. Pelvic MR undoubtedly offers beautiful depiction of myomas, is less operator-dependent compared with sonography, and produces reproducible images in standardized planes for

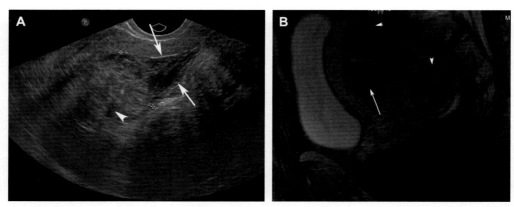

Fig. 9. A 39-year-old woman who had a history of myomas, post uterine artery embolization and vaginal bleeding. (*A*) Endovaginal sonography of the uterus, sagittal image, shows a well-defined mass with areas of shadowing (*arrowhead*) distorting the endometrial stripe. Complex fluid is present within the lower endometrial cavity compatible with blood (*arrows*). (*B*) Sagittal T2-weighted MR confirms the presence of a large submucosal myoma (*arrow*). Multiple intramural myomas are also present (*arrowheads*).

follow-up. MR may prove particularly advantageous if the uterus is large, with a volume exceeding 375 cm³, or if more than four myomas are present [14]. In a recently published study by Spielmann and colleagues [15], pelvic MR altered management in 11 of 49 women evaluated before UAE.

Significance of myoma enlargement over time

Many women who have known myomas undergo periodic pelvic sonograms to assess potential change in their size. Because their growth is estrogen-dependent, myomas can enlarge during pregnancy, in women who have anovulatory cycles, or in women undergoing tamoxifen therapy. They can also enlarge significantly during the fifth decade of life [1]. A rapid increase in size of myoma,

especially in young nonpregnant women or postmenopausal women, has been a traditional indication for hysterectomy in light of the potential for an underlying sarcomatous change. In a recent article entitled "Malignant transformation of myomas: myth or reality," Schwartz and Kelly [16] surmise that rapid growth not associated with vaginal bleeding or pain is not usually associated with malignancy and such patients can be managed conservatively.

Differential diagnosis

The diagnosis of uterine myomas is generally straightforward unless they are in an unusual location. The most common diagnostic dilemma is to differentiate between a myoma and adenomyosis, because both conditions are common.

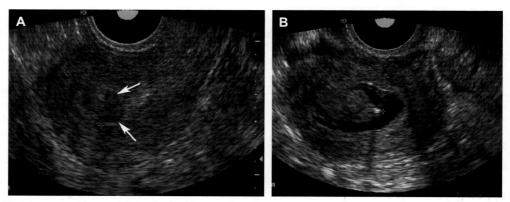

Fig. 10. A 51-year-old woman who had a history of myomas and vaginal bleeding. (*A*) Endovaginal sonography of the uterus, sagittal image, shows a hypoechoic mass within the endometrial cavity (*white arrows*). (*B*) Hysterosonography, coronal image, shows the mass outlined by fluid. Note the small calcification within the mass.

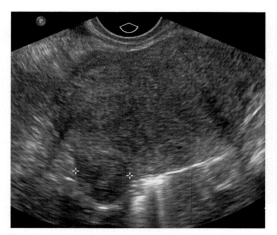

Fig. 11. A 40-year-old woman who had a history of enlarged uterus. Endovaginal sonography of the uterus, sagittal image, shows a small fundal subserosal myoma.

The sonographic appearance of adenomyosis is addressed in detail later. Table 1 describes the main sonographic features of each condition. As discussed earlier, a pedunculated myoma in the broad ligament can be mistaken for a solid ovarian mass, unless the ipsilateral ovary is clearly imaged. Ovarian fibromas, benign solid tumors of the ovary composed histologically of connective tissue, collagen, and stromal cells, have an echotexture similar to myomas (Fig. 15). Endometrial polyps and submucosal myomas present with mass effect on the endometrium. Color Doppler sonography or sonohysterography may depict multiple vessels arising from the myometrium feeding the submucosal myoma. By contrast, endometrial polyps are usually supplied by a single feeding vessel [17]. Occasionally a degenerating myoma containing cystic spaces mimics a missed abortion, a molar pregnancy, or even a cornual ectopic pregnancy.

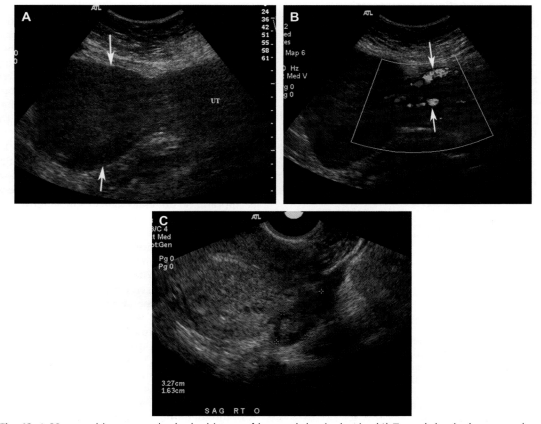

Fig. 12. A 33-year-old woman who had a history of lower abdominal pain. (*A*) Transabdominal sonography of the uterus, transverse image, shows a large hypoechoic mass in the right adnexa (*white arrows*) with a broad attachment to the uterus (UT). (*B*) On the transabdominal color Doppler transverse image, large blood vessels are extending from the uterine body to the mass (*arrows*). (*C*) Endovaginal sonography of the right adnexa, sagittal image, shows a normal, separate right ovary (between calipers). A 13-cm right pedunculated myoma was confirmed at surgery and was excised.

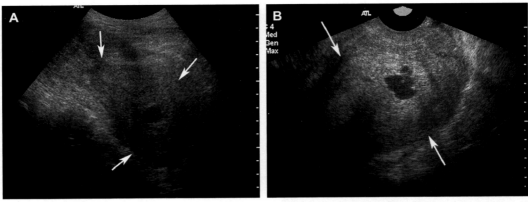

Fig. 13. A 36-year-old woman who had a history of vaginal bleeding and lower abdominal pain. (*A*) Transabdominal sonography of the lower uterus, sagittal image, shows a large heterogeneous mass distending the cervix (*arrows*). (*B*) On the endovaginal sagittal image, the borders of the mass (*arrows*) are not well seen. The patient underwent an abdominal hysterectomy and the diagnosis of a large myoma prolapsing through the cervix was confirmed.

Adenomyosis

Definition and clinical symptoms

Adenomyosis is a common disorder characterized by the presence of ectopic endometrial glands and

stroma within the myometrium, associated with hypertrophy of the adjacent smooth muscle fibers (Fig. 16). This disorder is a poorly demarcated infiltrative process that can diffusely involve the entire uterus or be more localized (Fig. 17). Pregnancy, cesarean section, dilatation and curettage, or other uterine trauma, along with chronic endometritis, cause disruption of the endometrial basal layer and may all be contributing factors to the development of adenomyosis. Another proposed mechanism is the migration of endometrial glands by way of vascular or lymphatic channels.

Adenomyosis has been reported in 5% to up to 70% of women in the fourth and fifth decade. This wide range is likely because this condition tended to be underdiagnosed, particularly before its appearance on endovaginal sonography and MR became widely recognized. Symptoms and signs are nonspecific and include dysfunctional uterine bleeding, menorrhagia, dysmenorrhea, and an enlarged, sometimes tender uterus. Although symptoms should abate after menopause because adenomyosis is estrogen-dependent, older women on tamoxifen may experience recrudescence of the disease. Awareness of the frequency of this condition and of its sometimes-subtle sonographic signs has lead to improved diagnostic accuracy. Imaging plays a critical role in women who have symptoms suggestive of adenomyosis. The ideal technique would allow not only accurate diagnosis of this condition but also reliable assessment of the severity of the condition, particularly the depth of myometrial extension. Finally, other conditions that may mimic adenomyosis, such as endometriosis, myomas, and dysfunctional uterine bleeding, need to be eliminated before surgical treatment is considered [18]. As discussed later, endovaginal

Table 1: **Sonographic diagnosis of uterine myoma and adenomyosis**

	Myoma	Adenomyosis
Uterus size	Variable normal to markedly enlarged	Normal to mildly enlarged
Uterus shape	Lobulated	Globular
Myometrium	Well defined mass Shadowing within the mass	Poorly defined heterogenous echotexture Scattered areas of shadowing Myometrial cysts Echogenic nodule Echogenic striations
Endometrial cavity	Well defined or distorted (submucous myoma) or Not clearly seen if many or large myomas	Poorly defined borders Subendometrial cysts
Color Doppler	A few feeding vessels surrounding the mass	Traversing vessels

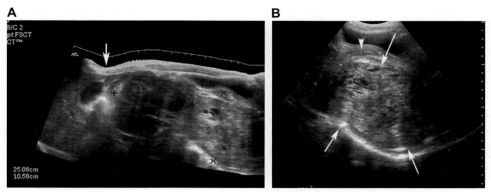

Fig. 14. A 35-year-old woman who had a history of 20-weeks' uterus on physical exam. (*A*) Transabdominal sonography of the lower abdomen with extended filed of view sagittal image shows a 25-cm uterus with multiple myomas. The fundus extends up to the patient's umbilicus (*arrow*). Note the multiple myomas. (*B*) Transabdominal sonography of the lower abdomen, sagittal image. The endometrial stripe is better seen on the conventional image (*arrowhead*). There is a large posterior heterogeneous myoma (*arrows*).

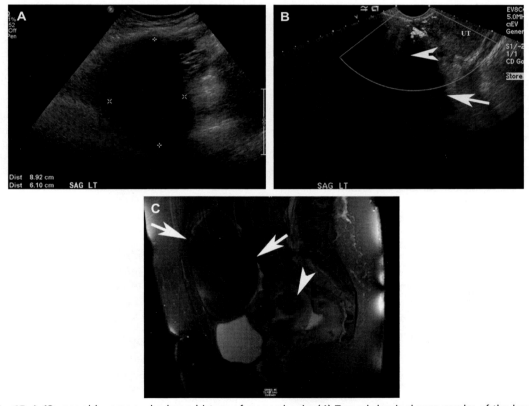

Fig. 15. A 43-year-old woman who has a history of menorrhagia. (*A*) Transabdominal sonography of the lower abdomen, sagittal image, shows a large markedly hypoechoic adnexal mass without distal acoustic enhancement. (*B*) Endovaginal sonography of the left adnexa with color Doppler, sagittal image, shows a partially visualized solid left adnexal mass (*arrow*) with acoustic shadowing (*arrowhead*). The left ovary could not be identified. Multiple uterine myomas were present (not shown). UT, uterus. (*C*) T2-weighted MR, sagittal image, shows the mass superior and to the left of the uterus (*arrows*) to have similar signal intensity to the uterine myomas (*arrowhead*). The mass displayed signal intensity and enhancement similar to myomas on T1-weighted sequence and after gadolinium injection (not shown). A large left ovarian fibroma was found at surgery.

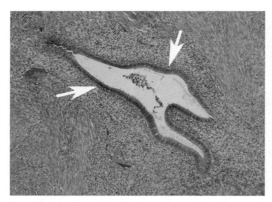

Fig. 16. Adenomyosis of the uterus, histology specimen. An endometrial gland (*arrows*) with adjacent stroma is embedded within the myometrium.

sonography has been shown to have high levels of sensitivity and specificity in experienced hands and should be the initial imaging modality in patients who have suspected adenomyosis. Pelvic MR is invaluable in equivocal or difficult cases [19].

Sonographic findings

A sonographic diagnosis of adenomyosis should be suggested when two or more of the following findings are present [20–22]. An elegant study by Atri and colleagues [23] correlated the histologic findings with sonographic appearance in 102 hysterectomy specimens.

> Globular shape of the uterine fundus without change in the contour of the uterus (Fig. 18)
> Heterogeneous mottled appearance of the myometrium, with asymmetric thickening and ill-defined echogenic areas within the myometrium. These areas are often elliptical in shape but produce no or minimal mass effect

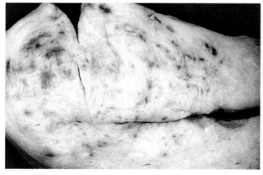

Fig. 17. Adenomyosis of the uterus, gross hysterectomy specimen. Extensive foci of adenomyosis are infiltrating the smooth muscle of the uterus. Note the absence of pseudocapsule.

(Fig. 19). Areas of increased echogenicity correspond to nests of endometrial glands. Scattered hypoechoic striations may also be present and correspond to smooth muscle hypertrophy (see Fig. 18).

> Small round echogenic nodules scattered within the uterine muscle (Fig. 20)
> Myometrial cysts, which correspond to cystically dilated endometrial glands. These are believed to be the most specific criterion for diagnosing adenomyosis (Fig. 21) [21].
> Poor definition of the endometrial stripe with pseudowidening of the endometrium (see Fig. 21)
> Echogenic striations radiating from the endometrial stripe (Fig. 22)

The sensitivity and specificity of sonography in the diagnosis of adenomyosis have been reported to reach 80% to 86% and 74% to 86%, respectively [22,24,25]. Atri and colleagues [23] found that subendometrial echogenic nodules, echogenic subendometrial striations, and asymmetric myometrial thickness had the best positive predictive value for the diagnosis. Many of the findings described here are subtle, easier to observe on real-time evaluation, and require meticulous scanning technique.

Adenomyotic cyst

Adenomyotic cyst is an uncommon manifestation of adenomyosis. It is produced by extensive and repeated menstrual bleeding within ectopic endometrial glands. On sonography, an adenomyotic cyst presents as a complex cystic mass filled with low-level echoes within the myometrium (Fig. 23). Subserosal, intramural, and submucosal locations have been described [26].

Differential diagnosis

The most common difficulty encountered in the diagnosis of uterine myometrial abnormalities is the differentiation between myomas and adenomyosis. Myomas tend to be overdiagnosed because the signs of adenomyosis can be subtle, unless they are sought for and observed in real time. Many reports describing "ill-defined myomas" in fact likely represent unrecognized adenomyosis. The difficulty is compounded by myomas and adenomyosis being common conditions that coexist in 36% to 50% of women (see Figs. 18 and 19) [22,27]. Some authors have emphasized the additional value of color or power Doppler in distinguishing the two entities. Myomas have one or two feeding vessels surrounding the mass, whereas vessels are freely traversing areas of adenomyosis without being displaced (Fig. 24) [20,28]. Differentiating

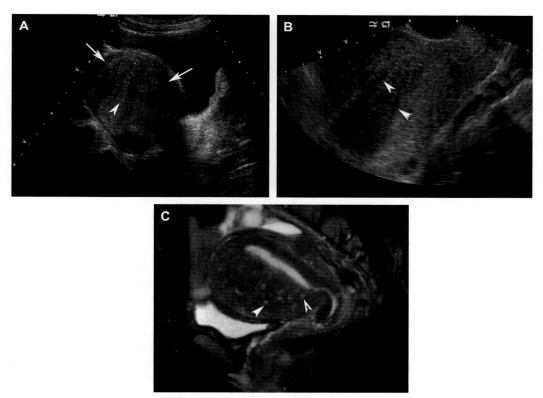

Fig. 18. A 48-year-old woman who had a history of lower abdominal pain. (*A*) Transabdominal sonography of the lower abdomen, sagittal image, shows a mildly enlarged uterus with bulky globular uterine fundus. Note heterogeneous echotexture of the thickened anterior myometrium (*arrows*), without discrete mass. There is a well-defined posterior myoma. Arrowhead indicates the endometrial stripe. (*B*) On the endovaginal sagittal image, hypoechoic striations in the anterior myometrium (*arrowheads*) are better depicted. (*C*) T2-weighted pelvic MR, sagittal reconstruction, shows thickening of the anterior junctional zone of the uterus with multiple high signal intensity foci, confirming the diagnosis of adenomyosis. Note the small posterior myoma.

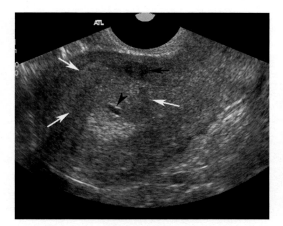

Fig. 19. A 42-year-old woman who had a history of pelvic pain and menorrhagia. Endovaginal ultrasound, sagittal image of the uterus shows an ill-defined echogenic area in a thickened anterior myometrium (*white arrows*). There is a small subendometrial cyst (*arrowhead*). Note the well-demarcated hypoechoic small myoma (*black arrow*). The diagnosis of adenomyosis was confirmed on the hysterectomy specimen.

between myomas and adenomyomas, a relatively well-circumscribed and focal form of adenomyosis, may be particularly challenging.

Limitation of sonography in the diagnosis of adenomyosis

Hysterectomy remains the traditional treatment of severe symptomatic adenomyosis. Recently, less invasive alternative therapies have become available. They include surgical endometrial ablation or resection and medical treatment with progestins, antigonadotropin danazol, and GnRH analogs. These treatments seem to be less effective against deep adenomyosis, however. One of the significant limitations of sonography is its limitation in assessing the depth of extension of adenomyosis within the myometrium and the severity of the process. Hulka and colleagues [27] have shown that the presence of myomas adversely affects the ability of endovaginal sonography to assess the severity of adenomyosis.

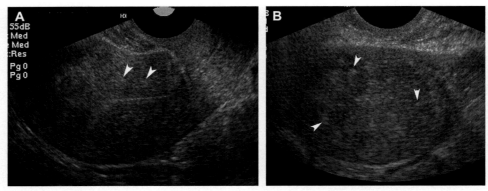

Fig. 20. A 45-year-old woman who had a history of menorrhagia and anemia. Endovaginal ultrasound, sagittal image (*A*) and coronal image (*B*) of the uterus shows a heterogeneous echotexture of the myometrium with multiple small echogenic foci scattered within the myometrium (*arrowheads*). The uterus is normal in size. The diagnosis of adenomyosis was confirmed on the hysterectomy specimen.

Pelvic MR has been shown to be more accurate in diagnosing adenomyosis in the presence of coexisting myomas and provides a more accurate estimation of the depth of myometrial invasion [19]. The role of pelvic MR is discussed later.

Uncommon myometrial tumors and tumorlike lesions

Fatty tumors

Fat-containing neoplasms of the uterus are rare benign tumors composed of a variable amount of mesenchymal tissue. They include lipomas, lipoleiomyomas, and fibromyolipomas. On sonography, the lesion is usually solitary and appears as a well-defined echogenic mass within the myometrium (Fig. 25). If the uterine origin of the mass is not recognized, the tumor may be mistaken for an ovarian cystic teratoma. Coexisting myomas can be present. If necessary, the diagnosis is easily confirmed by CT or MR [29].

Leiomyosarcoma and other malignant tumors of the myometrium

Uterine sarcomas, malignant tumors of mesodermal origins, are much less common than endometrial carcinoma, representing only 2% to 6% of uterine cancer. They include leiomyosarcomas, malignant mixed mesodermal tumors (MMMT), and rarer neoplasms, such as endometrial stromal sarcomas and rhabdomyosarcomas. Leiomyosarcomas are the most common histologic type of uterine sarcoma. They are rarely diagnosed preoperatively. Malignant mixed mesodermal tumors contain sarcomatous elements and foci of carcinomas Reviews of large numbers of hysterectomy

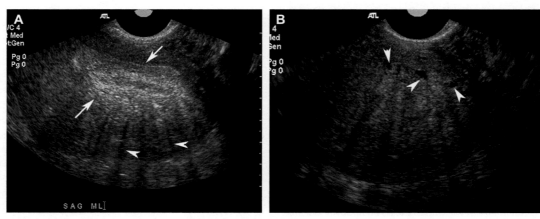

Fig. 21. A 42-year-old woman who had a history of menorrhagia. (*A*) Endovaginal ultrasound, sagittal image of the uterus shows poor definitions of the borders of the endometrial stripe (*arrows*). There are hypoechoic striations within the myometrium (*arrowheads*). The uterus is retroverted. (*B*) Endovaginal ultrasound, sagittal image of the myometrium shows several small myometrial cysts (*arrowheads*). This patient elected management with medical therapy.

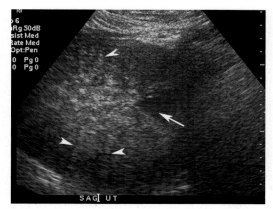

Fig. 22. A 56-year-old woman who had a history of menorrhagia and uterine enlargement. Transabdominal sonography of the uterine fundus, sagittal image shows a globular shape with echogenic striations radiating from the region of the endometrial stripe (*arrowheads*). There is a myometrial cyst (*arrow*). The hysterectomy specimen demonstrated extensive adenomyosis.

specimens have shown that the incidence of unsuspected sarcomas associated with myomas is estimated at 0.13% to 0.49% [30]. Uterine sarcomas, particularly MMMT, tend to manifest themselves after menopause [31]. The possibility of an underlying sarcoma should be raised in an older woman who has a rapidly enlarging myoma, particularly if there is associated vaginal bleeding. The sonographic appearance of uterine sarcomas is that of a large uterine mass with heterogeneous echotexture and areas of cystic necrosis (**Figs. 26 and 27**). Several series have shown that leiomyosarcomas cannot be reliably differentiated from the far more common myomas on gray-scale sonography.

The presence of abdominal adenopathy or masses in an older woman should raise the specter of uterine malignancy (see **Fig. 26**). Although some authors speculate that Doppler sonography may be helpful, these studies are limited by the small number of patients [32]. Endometrial carcinoma is the most common malignant tumor of the uterine corpus, and arises from the endometrium, but diagnosis of secondary extension into the myometrium is critical for patient management. Accurate estimation of the depth of myometrial invasion has important prognostic implications because nodal metastases are six to seven times more likely in the presence of myometrial extension of 50% or greater. In a patient who has endometrial cancer, myometrial invasion should be suspected if there is a disruption of the subendometrial halo and heterogeneous echotexture of the myometrium adjacent to the thickened endometrium. Coexistent adenomyosis may mimic myometrial invasion, however, and it has been shown that contrast-enhanced MR is more accurate than endovaginal ultrasound in predicting depth of invasion [33].

Effect of tamoxifen therapy on the myometrium

Tamoxifen citrate is a selective estrogen receptor modulator widely used for the treatment and prevention of breast cancer. Contrary to its antiestrogen effect on the breast, it acts as an estrogen agonist on the postmenopausal endometrium and myometrium. Women taking tamoxifen undergo regular vaginal sonograms to monitor endometrial thickness and detect developing endometrial hyperplasia, polyps, and carcinoma. Enlargement of myomas and reactivation of foci of adenomyosis

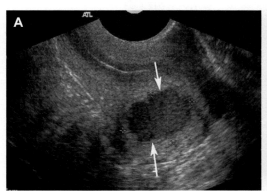
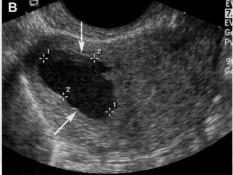

Fig. 23. An 18-year-old woman who had a history of pelvic pain. (*A*) Endovaginal ultrasound, sagittal image of the uterus shows a cyst filled with low-level echoes within the myometrium (*arrows*). The uterus is retroverted. (*B*) Endovaginal ultrasound, coronal image of the myometrium confirmed the finding (*arrows*). Pelvic MR and ultrasound guided aspiration of this lesion were consistent with old blood (not shown). This myometrial mass was subsequently excised; the pathologic diagnosis was an adenomyoma.

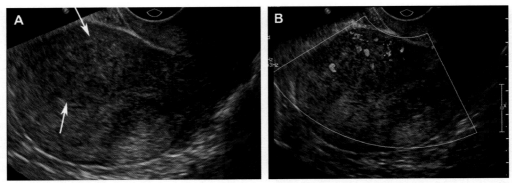

Fig. 24. A 47-year-old woman who had a history of vaginal bleeding. (*A*) Endovaginal ultrasound, sagittal image of the uterus shows an ill-defined region of heterogeneous echotexture in the anterior myometrium (*arrows*). (*B*) Endovaginal ultrasound, sagittal image of the uterus with color Doppler shows myometrial vessels freely coursing to this region, favoring the diagnosis of adenomyosis.

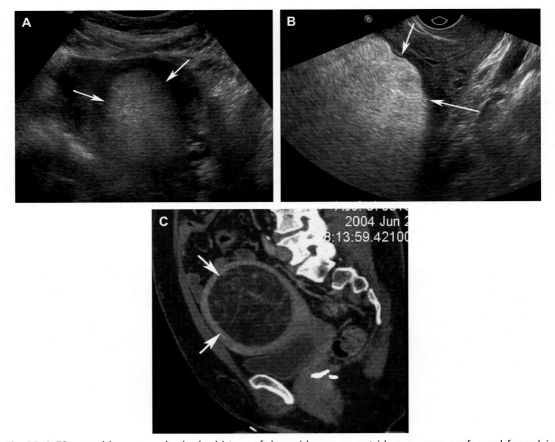

Fig. 25. A 58-year-old woman who had a history of dermoid seen on outside sonogram performed for pelvic cramps. (*A*) Transabdominal sonography of the uterus, transverse image, shows a well-defined echogenic mass within the uterus (*arrows*). No separate adnexal mass was present. (*B*) Endovaginal ultrasound, sagittal image of the uterus confirms that the echogenic mass (*arrows*) is indeed arising within the uterus. (*C*) Unenhanced CT, sagittal reconstruction shows a uterine fatty mass (*arrows*). Hysterectomy specimen yielded a 12-cm lipoleiomyoma.

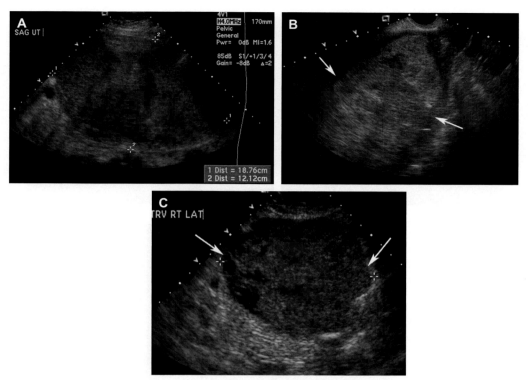

Fig. 26. A 68-year-old woman who had a history of postmenopausal bleeding and a negative endometrial biopsy. (*A*) Transabdominal sonography of the uterus, sagittal image, shows an enlarged uterus with heterogeneous echotexture. The endometrial stripe cannot be identified. (*B*) Endovaginal ultrasound, sagittal image of the uterus shows a heterogeneous mass in the uterus (*arrows*). The endometrial stripe is not seen. The sonographic appearance is concerning for endometrial cancer with myometrial invasion or myometrial cancer. (*C*) Transabdominal ultrasound of the right flank shows a soft tissue mass within the abdomen (*arrows*). Many other abdominal masses were present, compatible with carcinomatosis. A high-grade uterine rhabdomyosarcoma with extensive abdominal metastases was found at surgery.

in postmenopausal women have been associated with tamoxifen therapy (Fig. 28) [34].

Uterine arteriovenous malformation

Uterine arteriovenous malformations are classified as congenital or acquired. The latter are much more common and usually follow a dilatation and curettage procedure. Iatrogenic trauma to the myometrium leads to the creation of single or multiple arteriovenous fistulae (AVF) between branches of myometrial arteries and veins. Women usually present with intermittent vaginal bleeding. Endovaginal sonography with color Doppler demonstrates a tangle of vessels with multidirectional flow creating a mosaic pattern. The diagnosis is confirmed by spectral Doppler finding of high-velocity high-diastolic turbulent arterial flow within the AVF. It should be emphasized, however, that the gray-scale appearance of these fistulas is subtle and consists of areas of heterogeneity within the myometrium or intramural cystic spaces representing the dilated

vessels (Fig. 29) [35]. Awareness of this diagnosis in patients who have vaginal bleeding, particularly if there is a history of prior uterine intervention, is essential to avoid a missed diagnosis. Many AVFs resolve spontaneously, but angiography followed by embolization is effective for treatment of intractable or life-threatening vaginal bleeding.

Role of pelvic MR imaging in evaluation of the myometrium

Diagnosis of leiomyomas

MR imaging is an excellent imaging modality to evaluate the female pelvis. Because of its superior soft tissue contrast resolution, MR imaging allows detailed assessment of the anatomy of the uterus, especially on T2-weighted images; the endometrial complex, junctional zone, myometrium, and serosal surface can be well visualized. This visualization becomes important in the evaluation of leiomyomas and adenomyosis. Multiplanar acquisition of

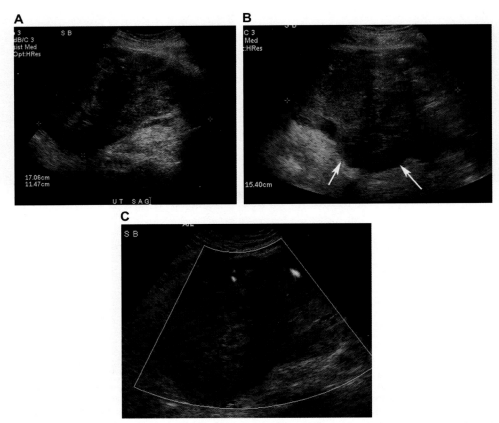

Fig. 27. A 65-year-old woman who had a history of postmenopausal bleeding and an enlarging pelvic mass. (*A*) Transabdominal sonography of the uterus, sagittal image, shows an enlarged uterus with heterogeneous echotexture. (*B*) Transabdominal sonography of the uterus, transverse image, confirms the findings and demonstrates lobulation of the uterine contour (*arrows*). (*C*) Transabdominal sonography of the uterus with power Doppler, sagittal image, shows minimal blood flow in the mass. Although the sonographic appearance is nonspecific and could be caused by myomas or sarcoma, it was believed that the age of the patient and particularly the history of enlarging pelvic mass were concerning. A pelvic MR was recommended; instead the patient underwent abdominal CT without contrast that showed retroperitoneal adenopathy and an enlarged uterus (not shown). An undifferentiated uterine sarcoma was found at pathology.

MR images improves the assessment of the uterine contour and the endometrial canal. Congenital Mullerian duct anomalies can thus be well assessed and anatomic relationships within the uterus (submucosal, intramural, subserosal localization of myomas) and between the uterus and adnexa can be defined. Soft tissue characterization with MR imaging based on tissue relaxation properties can be performed to identify fibrous tissue, hemorrhage, or fat containing uterine pathologies. Because of its cost and more limited availability, MR imaging is generally indicated as a problem-solving technique for various gynecologic disorders. It is much less operator-dependent than sonography, allows multiplanar imaging at larger field of view to define the precise anatomical location, and acquires reproducible images in standardized planes that facilitate follow-up. MR imaging allows: (1) differentiating pedunculated or contour-deforming myomas from adnexal masses; (2) mapping the number, size, and location of fibroids before and after therapy; (3) differentiating between myomas and adenomyosis; (4) characterizing tissue composition of myomas; (5) assessing myomas supplied by parasitized ovarian arteries; and (6) predicting the therapy response of myomas not only to the UAE but also to GnRH analog.

Subserosal pedunculated leiomyomas may pose diagnostic dilemma on EVS because they may appear to be adnexal masses if their site of origin from the uterus is not visualized. On MR imaging, typical leiomyomas are of low signal intensity on T2-weighted sequences because of their composition of smooth muscle with varying amounts of

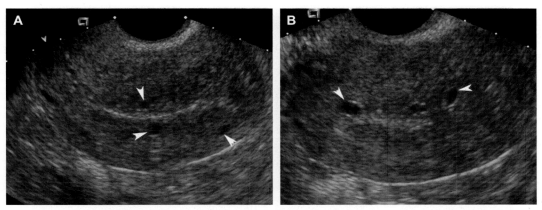

Fig. 28. A 64-year-old woman who had a history of tamoxifen therapy for 4 years. Endovaginal ultrasound, sagittal image (*A*) and coronal image (*B*) of the uterus shows a heterogeneous echotexture of the myometrium with multiple small myometrial and subendometrial cysts (*arrowheads*) consistent with adenomyosis.

fibrous connective tissue [36]. The main feature that increases specificity of diagnosis of exophytic leiomyomas with MR imaging is the ability to define the origin of the adnexal mass from the uterus, a stalklike connection to the uterus, or the presence of a bridging vascular sign representing tortuous vascular structures crossing between the uterus and the leiomyoma (Fig. 30) [37,38]. This finding is best seen on T2-weighted images and gadolinium-enhanced T1-weighted images; the vessels

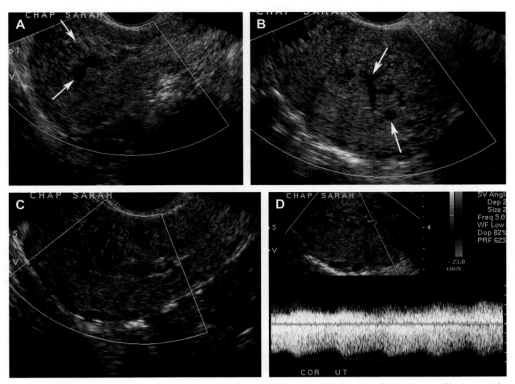

Fig. 29. A 28-year-old woman who had a history of persistent vaginal bleeding following a dilation and curettage. (*A*) Endovaginal ultrasound, sagittal image of the lateral uterus, shows small cystic spaces in the myometrium (*arrows*). The endometrial stripe was minimally thickened (not shown). (*B*) The coronal endovaginal image confirms the finding. (*C*) Sagittal endovaginal image of the uterus with color Doppler shows the cystic spaces in the myometrium correspond to a tangle of vessels. (*D*) The Doppler spectrum confirms the presence of an arteriovenous fistula as evidenced by turbulent low-resistance flow within these vessels. The diagnosis was confirmed on contrast-enhanced MR.

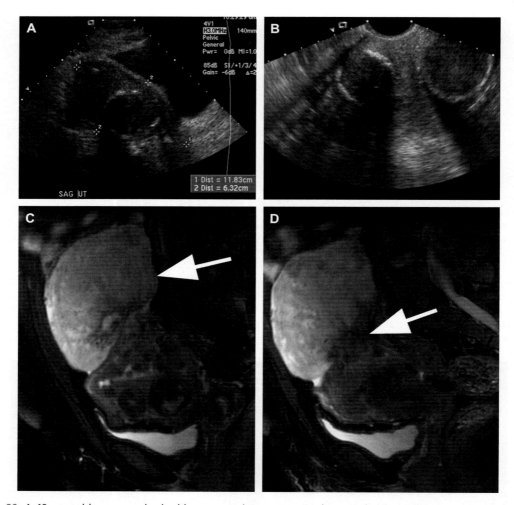

Fig. 30. A 49-year-old woman who had known uterine myomas and new enlarging pelvic mass. Hysterectomy showed a cellular 11-cm leiomyoma composed of spindle cells showing mild cytologic atypia and apparent smooth differentiation. There was no significant mitotic activity. Ultrasound showed a predominantly solid mass with cystic areas superior to the fundus, not visualized on US examination 4 years before. Mass was believed to represent exophytic degenerating fibroid versus predominantly solid ovarian carcinoma. Pelvic MR imaging was recommended for further characterization. (*A*) TAS sagittal view of the uterus shows moderate enlargement attributable to fibroids. (*B*) Endovaginal coronal image of the uterus shows bilateral circumscribed masses with peripheral echogenic rim of calcification, compatible with fibroids. (*C*) MR imaging, sagittal T2-weighted image (TR/TE 3616/77ms) shows bulky uterus with multiple fibroids and a large exophytic mass arising from the posterior fundal myometrium (*arrow*). Mass shows T2 bright signal compatible with high cellular composition. (*D*) MR imaging sagittal T2-weighted image shows a stalk of myometrial tissue between the myometrium and the exophytic mass (*arrow*). (*E*) MR imaging, axial T2-weighted image (TR/TE 4566/84 ms) shows T2 dark signal of the well-circumscribed fibroids (*arrows*). (*F*) MR imaging axial T2-weighted image shows myomas in submucosal (*arrowhead*) and exophytic subserosal location (*arrow*). (*G*) MR imaging axial T2-weighted image shows a cellular fundal myoma with high signal intensity (*white arrow*) and bilateral areas of cystic degeneration (*arrowheads*). Note vascular bridge presenting as signal voids (*black arrow*). (*H*) MR imaging axial T1-weighted image shows T1 bright tubular signal in the region of vascular bridging vessels with slow flow (*arrow*). Vascular bridge is a sign of a vascular pedicle in an exophytic uterine mass. (*I*) MR imaging, axial T1-weighted image (TR/TE 600/20 ms) shows peripheral signal voids in hyalinized myomas with peripheral calcification (*arrows*). (*J*) MR imaging coronal T1-weighted GRE image (TR/TE 225/1.0 ms) after contrast administration shows nonenhancing fibroids (*arrows*) with peripheral rim of signal void compatible with calcifications corresponding to US in Fig. 1. Lack of contrast enhancement within calcified myomas is compatible with hyalinized degeneration. (*K*) MR imaging coronal T1-weighted GRE image after contrast at the level of exophytic mass shows avid enhancement of cellular fibroid (*arrow*) and lack of enhancement in the areas of cystic degeneration (*arrowheads*).

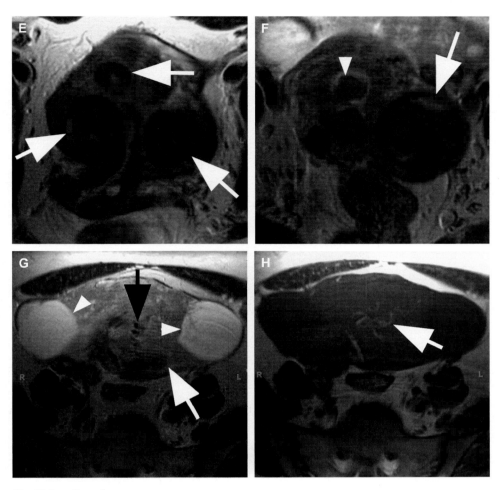

Fig. 30 (*continued*)

appear as curvilinear tortuous signal voids (see Fig. 30). Compared with pelvic MR imaging, color Doppler ultrasound has the added advantage of showing either arterial or venous blood flow signals between or crossing the uterus and the subserous leiomyoma [39]. Fibroids can also arise from the extrauterine structures, such as broad ligament or round ligament. Most of these extrauterine myomas have tissue characteristics typical of fibroids, T2 dark signal, and can be easily diagnosed with MR imaging, which also shows good definition of ovaries separate from those masses. Subserosal and extrauterine myomas can acquire vascularity from ovarian arteries. Contrast-enhanced MR angiography can help predict ovarian artery supply of uterine fibroids [40]. Most myomas grow slowly, and some remain relatively unchanged over prolonged periods. As leiomyomas enlarge, they may outgrow their blood supply, resulting in various types of degeneration (see Fig. 30). The diagnosis

of a degenerating myoma should be considered in a patient who has known fibroids and an acute onset of pelvic pain. The patient can also develop fever and an elevated white blood cell count (without a left shift) that can be confused with infection. Cystic degeneration of myoma can sometimes lead to a complex and confusing appearance on EVS but can be well characterized with MR imaging (Fig. 31). Rapid growth (eg, in pregnant patients) can lead to a hemorrhagic infarction (red degeneration) resulting in foci of high signal on T1- and T2-weighted images (Fig. 32). Red degeneration occurs secondary to venous thrombosis within the periphery of the tumor or rupture of intratumoral arteries [41]. In the past, rapid growth was considered worrisome for leiomyosarcoma. Parker and colleagues [42] showed, however, that incidence of uterine sarcoma (leiomyosarcoma, endometrial stromal sarcoma, and mixed mesodermal tumor) among patients who had rapidly enlarging uterine

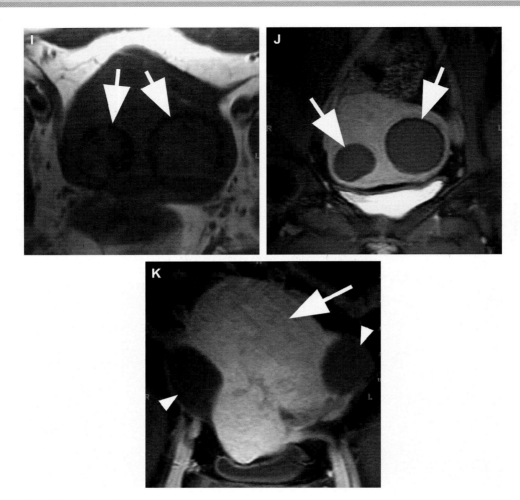

Fig. 30 (*continued*)

leiomyoma was extremely low (0.27%) and that the risk for developing a leiomyosarcoma was identical to that in stable myomas (0.21%). Rapid growth in postmenopausal women should be treated with greater caution, however. The distinction between a leiomyoma and a leiomyosarcoma cannot be reliably made on MR imaging. With the evidence of extrauterine extension, lymphadenopathy and metastases malignancy should be suspected.

Leiomyomas with intermediate to increased signal intensity on T2-weighted MR images correlate with the increased cellularity and proliferative activity of leiomyomas (see *Fig. 30*) and with good tumor response to UAE and GnRH analog treatment [43,44]. GnRH analog treatment may make myomas less discrete on imaging and may even make removal of fibroids more difficult. It was shown by Deligdisch and colleagues [45] in a histologic study that the cleavage planes between the myoma and the myometrium in hysterectomy

specimens was lost in 91% of patients pretreated with GnRH analogs.

Role of MR imaging in treatment planning of myomas

In the United States, women considering UAE often undergo pelvic MR imaging for preprocedure planning. MRI can provide accurate information on the size, location and soft tissue composition of myomas and allows mulitplanar imaging at larger field of view to define the precise anatomical location (*Fig. 33*).

Preprocedure imaging is essential for appropriate patient selection because the most important deciding factors include the size and location of the tumors [12]. UAE is most beneficial for intramural myomas. Purely submucosal lesions are best removed surgically; however partially submucosal myomas have been shown to respond well to UAE [46], with a significantly greater reduction in

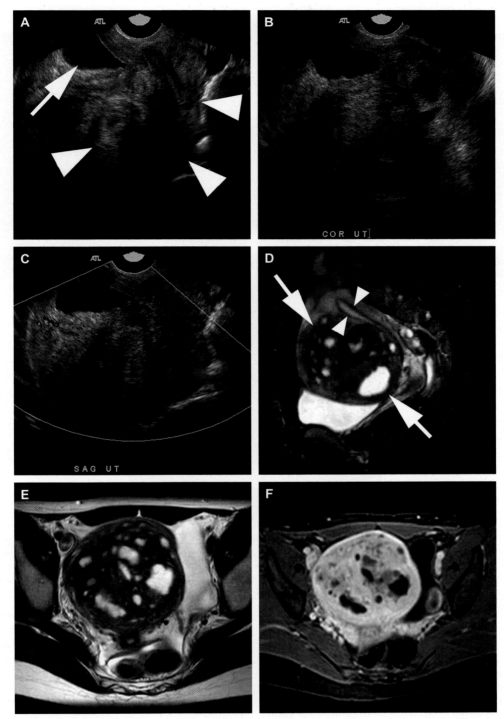

Fig. 31. A 30-year-old woman presenting with pelvic pain and a large fibroid with cystic degeneration. (*A*) Endovaginal sonogram, sagittal view of the uterus shows heterogeneous myometrium (*arrowheads*) with striations and large cystic spaces (*arrow*). (*B*) Endovaginal sonogram, coronal view, shows heterogeneity of myometrium, cystic areas, and non-visualization of discrete margins. (*C*) Endovaginal sonogram with color Doppler sagittal image of the uterus image shows nonspecific vascular pattern. (*D*) MR imaging, sagittal T2-weighted image (R/TE 3721/70 ms), shows T2-dark mass with visible margins and cystic areas (*arrows*) separate from the normal junctional zone (*arrowheads*). Visualization of the normal junctional zone rules out adenomyosis. (*E*) MR imaging axial T2-weighted image (TR/TE 3500/90 ms) shows T2-dark mass with numerous internal T2-bright cystic foci. (*F*) MR imaging axial T1-weighted GRE image after contrast (TR/TE 4.1/2 ms) shows avid enhancement of the myoma except for areas of cystic degeneration.

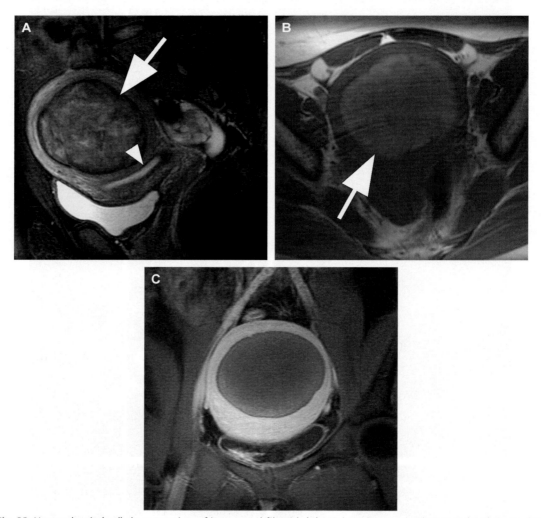

Fig. 32. Hemorrhagic (red) degeneration of intramural fibroid. (*A*) MR imaging, sagittal T2-weighted image (TR/TE 3473/70 ms), shows a circumscribed intramural mass (*arrow*) with well-defined margins and increased internal signal. Mass is separate from the junctional zone (*arrowhead*). (*B*) MR imaging, axial T1-weighted image (TR/TE 660/14 ms), shows T1-bright signal within the mass, compatible with hemorrhage (*arrow*). (*C*) MR imaging, coronal T1-weighted GRE image after contrast (TR/TE 4.1/2 ms), shows a complete lack of enhancement within the degenerated fibroid.

volume after UAE as compared with the reduction associated with an intramural or subserosal leiomyoma. Pedunculated myomas with limited attachment to the uterine body are not typically treated with UAE because of the risk for stalk infarction and subsequent detachment of the mass from the uterus and peritoneal irritation [12]. It has been reported, however, that subserosal myomas with the attachment greater than 2 cm can respond well to UAE without complications [47]. Contrast enhancement of leiomyomas as evaluated on MR imaging can predict their response to therapy: avidly enhancing myomas are best responders and nonenhancing myomas are nonresponders.

Calcified myomas or myomas with cystic or hemorrhagic degeneration and poor vascular supply respond less than optimally to embolization [13]. Nonviable leiomyomas are present in 20% of patients referred for UAE. In approximately two thirds of these patients, these nonviable leiomyomas are not dominant, and would not preclude UAE. If the dominant myomas are nonviable, however, this precludes UAE because these lesions lack blood flow at baseline [48]. Hyaline degeneration of fibroids is the expected result of treatment; however, some fibroids present at baseline as hyalinized leiomyomas that have low signal intensities on T2-weighted images similar to those of ordinary

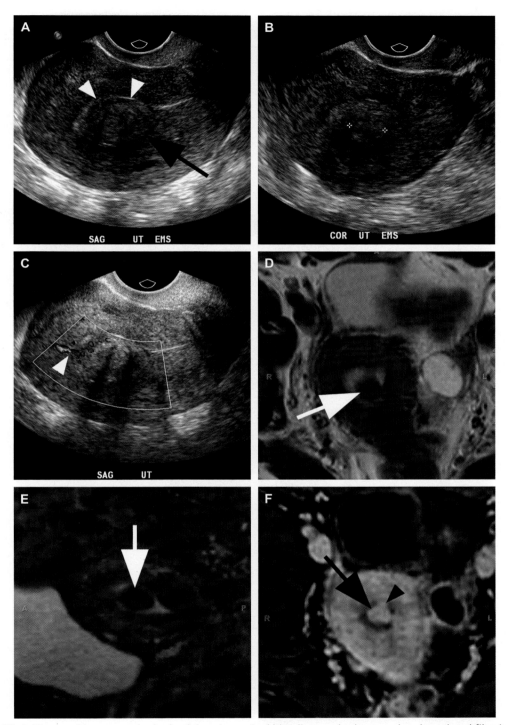

Fig. 33. A 48-year-old woman who had pelvic pain, vaginal bleeding, and submucosal pedunculated fibroid suspected on US and confirmed on MR imaging. (*A*) Endovaginal sonography, sagittal view of the uterus shows a small heterogeneous mass (*arrow*) with striations distorting the endometrial complex (*arrowheads*). (*B*) Endovaginal sonography, coronal view shows a discrete submucosal mass. (*C*) Endovaginal sonography, color Doppler image shows a feeding vessel to the mass (*arrowhead*). (*D*) MR imaging, axial T2-weighted image (TR/TE 3500/90 ms), shows a small, circumscribed mass on a stalk projecting into the endometrial canal (*arrow*). (*E*) MR imaging, sagittal T2-weighted image (TR/TE 3473/70 ms), shows T2 dark signal of the mass typical for of the submucosal fibroid (*arrow*). (*F*) MR imaging, axial T2-weighted GRE image (TR/TE 4.1/2 ms) after contrast administration, shows intense enhancement of fibroid (*arrow*) similar to that of myometrium. Note enhancement of the stalk (*arrowhead*).

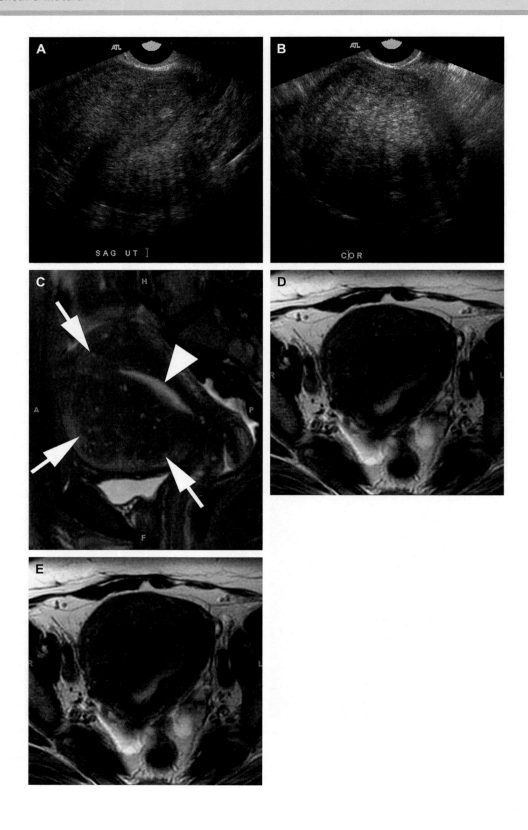

leiomyomas. Completely hyalinized leiomyomas show little enhancement and thus can be differentiated from ordinary leiomyomas on dynamic contrast-enhanced MR imaging (see Fig. 30). Successful medical treatment with GnRH analogs or UAE cannot be expected for hyalinized myomas, because they are already in the hyalinized state that is the goal of therapy and further reduction in size would not take place [49].

Role of MR imaging in the diagnosis of adenomyosis

The importance of MR imaging in diagnosis of adenomyosis has been documented [50]. The subendometrial myometrium, which is composed of closely packed muscle cells, is easily visualized by MR imaging as a low signal intensity zone, the junctional zone, on T2-weighted images, [51]. Although endovaginal sonography can demonstrate findings suggestive of adenomyosis, the soft tissue definition provided by MR imaging allows specific identification of the thickening of the junctional zone, which is nonuniform and usually not well-demarcated, with T1 and T2 bright foci representing heterotopic endometrium, cystic dilatation of heterotopic glands (Fig. 34), or hemorrhagic foci characterizing adenomyosis. Adenomyosis can present as a localized process with a masslike focal thickening of the junctional zone (adenomyoma) or a diffuse process involving the large portion of the myometrium (see Fig. 34; Figs. 35 and 36). Contrast enhancement in MR imaging does not add significantly to a diagnosis of adenomyosis, because it is an infiltrative process with heterogeneous enhancement, which is nonspecific. The sensitivity and specificity of MR imaging in the diagnosis of adenomyosis has been shown to be superior to that of endovaginal sonography: sensitivity of MR imaging 0.70 (95% CI, 0.46–0.87) and EVS 0.68 (95% CI, 0.44–0.86); specificity of MR imaging 0.86 (95% CI, 0.76–0.93) and EVS 0.65 (95% CI, 0.50–0.77) [52]. A laparoscopy-guided myometrial biopsy in the diagnosis of diffuse adenomyosis has been recently proposed [53]. MR imaging allows noninvasive assessment of adenomyosis and its extent alleviating the need for interventional diagnostic procedures. Other advantages of MR over sonography include improved diagnosis of adenomyosis in patients who have coexisting myomas (see Fig. 36) and better triaging for women considering less invasive treatments for adenomyosis.

Compared with sonography, MR imaging allows better assessment of the depth of extension of adenomyosis within the myometrium and the severity of the process. This information is critical for women who have symptomatic adenomyosis who elect to preserve their uterus. Endometrial ablation or resection is less effective against deep adenomyosis; therefore the extent of adenomyosis (eg, focal [adenomyoma] versus diffuse, mild superficial versus deep infiltrative) as defined on MR images can guide best management. Although MR imaging is highly accurate in differentiating adenomyosis from leiomyomas, the imaging characteristics may overlap, especially in the case of adenomyoma. Features that favor the diagnosis of adenomyosis include a mass with poorly defined borders (when myoma shows circumscribed, well-defined margins), minimal mass effect on the endometrium relative to the size of lesion, continuity with the junctional zone, linear striations radiating from endometrium to myometrium, and presence of high-signal foci.

Controversy exists regarding the effectiveness of UAE in the management of symptomatic adenomyosis. Recent results indicate that UAE is effective in the management of symptomatic adenomyosis and has an acceptable long-term success rate [54]. MR imaging can be used before and after UAE therapy to monitor treatment effect. The recurrence rate associated with UAE for isolated adenomyosis is higher than that for treatment of uterine fibroid tumors, because vascularization in diffuse adenomyosis (in which smaller arteries extend throughout the myometrium) is different from that in fibroids that have feeding vessels [55]. It has been hypothesized that embolization with the use of large particles may not be effective for treating adenomyosis. The use of small particles, although appearing more effective, may also cause injury to normal tissue. Appropriate diagnosis of adenomyosis is therefore important at the time of

Fig. 34. A 49-year-old woman who had menometrorrhagia and adenomyosis. (*A*) Endovaginal sonography, sagittal view, shows heterogeneous myometrium with striations. (*B*) Endovaginal sonography, coronal view, shows that there is no discrete mass within the heterogeneous myometrium. (*C*) MR imaging, sagittal T2-weighted image (TR/TE 5200/83 ms), shows marked thickening of the junctional zone, which has irregular margins, scattered bright foci typical for a diffuse adenomyosis (*arrows*). Note that the infiltrated anterior myometrium is asymmetrically thicker than the posterior. Endometrial complex (*arrowhead*). (*D*) MR imaging, axial T2-weighted image (TR/TE 3566/120 ms), shows continuity of the dark signal replacing the right anterolateral myometrium with the junctional zone. No discrete margins can be outlined. (*E*) MR imaging, axial T1-weighted GRE image (TR/TE 5.3/2.3 ms) after contrast administration, shows heterogeneous enhancement of myometrium without a discrete mass.

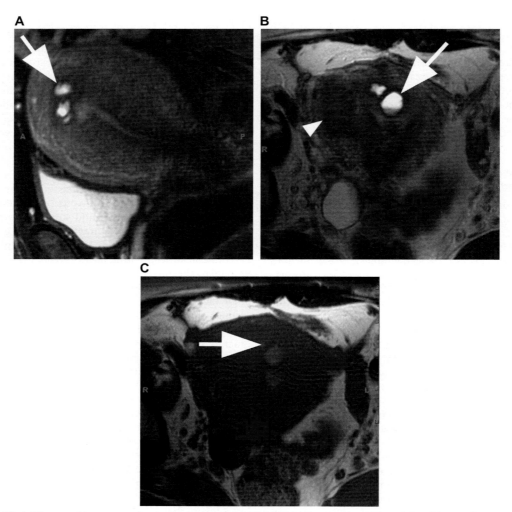

Fig. 35. A 38-year-old woman who had adenomyosis. (*A*) MR imaging, sagittal T2-weighted image (TR/TE 4200/77 ms), shows thickening of the junctional zone greater than 15 mm with cystic endometrial implants (*arrow*). (*B*) MR imaging, axial T2-weighted image (TR/TE 4400/121 ms), shows cystic areas within the thickened junctional zone (*arrow*). Note right intramural fibroid with T2 dark signal (*arrowhead*). (*C*) MR imaging, axial T2-weighted image (TR/TE 416/9 ms), shows T1 bright signal of hemorrhage within the endometrial implants (*arrow*).

the initial evaluation. MR imaging with its superior accuracy to detect adenomyosis is the preferred imaging modality for baseline assessment, even though EVS, when augmented with CDUS, may demonstrate characteristic multiple scattered vessels or internal irregular vascularity in adenomyosis without a dominant feeding or surrounding vessel that is typical for a myoma.

Summary

Pelvic sonography remains the imaging modality of choice for initial evaluation of myometrial pathology. The advent of vaginal sonography and color Doppler sonography have allowed for major refinements in detection and accurate diagnoses of common disorders affecting the uterus, particularly myomas and adenomyosis.

Pelvic MR imaging undoubtedly plays an important role in gynecologic imaging because it depicts details of myometrium and junctional zone, is more reproducible, and is less operator-dependent when compared with sonography. Because of its higher cost and lesser availability, MR imaging is usually reserved for pretreatment planning and for problem solving in patients for whom the ultrasound is inconclusive, not feasible, or technically suboptimal.

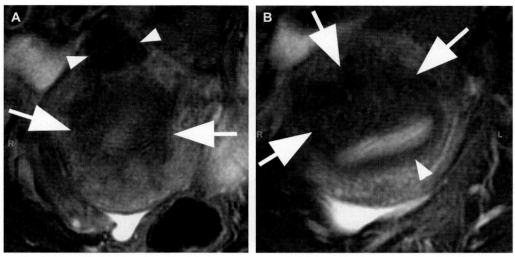

Fig. 36. A 39-year-old woman who had menorrhagia and pelvic pain, adenomyosis and fibroid. (*A*) MR imaging, axial T2-weighted image (TR/TE 3616/77 ms) of the uterus shows irregular thickening of the junctional zone (*arrows*) compatible with adenomyosis. Note circumscribed low-intensity myoma anteriorly (*arrowheads*). (*B*) MR imaging, axial T2-weighted image, shows focal masslike T2-dark signal abnormality continuous with the junctional zone (*arrows*) compatible with adenomyoma. Note normal thickness of the intact posterior junctional zone (*arrowhead*).

References

[1] Wallach EE, Vlahos NF. Uterine myomas: an overview of development, clinical features, and management. Obstet Gynecol 2004;104(2):393–406.

[2] Kjerulff KH, et al. Uterine leiomyomas. Racial differences in severity, symptoms and age at diagnosis. J Reprod Med 1996;41(7):483–90.

[3] Cramer SF, Patel A. The frequency of uterine leiomyomas. Am J Clin Pathol 1990;94(4):435–8.

[4] Becker E Jr, et al. The added value of transvaginal sonohysterography over transvaginal sonography alone in women with known or suspected leiomyoma. J Ultrasound Med 2002;21(3):237–47.

[5] Tulandi T. Treatment of uterine fibroids—is surgery obsolete? N Engl J Med 2007;356(4):411–3.

[6] Karasick S, Lev-Toaff AS, Toaff ME. Imaging of uterine leiomyomas. AJR Am J Roentgenol 1992; 158(4):799–805.

[7] Caoili EM, et al. Refractory shadowing from pelvic masses on sonography: a useful diagnostic sign for uterine leiomyomas. AJR Am J Roentgenol 2000;174(1):97–101.

[8] Cohen LS, Valle RF. Role of vaginal sonography and hysterosonography in the endoscopic treatment of uterine myomas. Fertil Steril 2000;73(2): 197–204.

[9] Tiltman AJ. Leiomyomas of the uterine cervix: a study of frequency. Int J Gynecol Pathol 1998;17(3):231–4.

[10] Varras M, et al. Clinical considerations and sonographic findings of a large nonpedunculated primary cervical leiomyoma complicated by heavy vaginal haemorrhage: a case report and review of the literature. Clin Exp Obstet Gynecol 2003; 30(2–3):144–6.

[11] Ravina JH, et al. Arterial embolisation to treat uterine myomata. Lancet 1995;346(8976):671–2.

[12] Pelage JP, Fauconnier A. Uterine fibroid embolization: where are we and where should we go? Ultrasound Obstet Gynecol 2005;25(6):527–34.

[13] Ghai S, et al. Uterine artery embolization for leiomyomas: pre- and postprocedural evaluation with US. Radiographics 2005;25(5):1159–72 [discussion: 1173–6].

[14] Dueholm M, et al. Accuracy of magnetic resonance imaging and transvaginal ultrasonography in the diagnosis, mapping, and measurement of uterine myomas. Am J Obstet Gynecol 2002; 186(3):409–15.

[15] Spielmann AL, et al. Comparison of MRI and sonography in the preliminary evaluation for fibroid embolization. AJR Am J Roentgenol 2006; 187(6):1499–504.

[16] Schwartz PE, Kelly MG. Malignant transformation of myomas: myth or reality? Obstet Gynecol Clin North Am 2006;33(1):183–98, xii.

[17] Fleischer AC, Shappell HW. Color Doppler sonohysterography of endometrial polyps and submucosal fibroids. J Ultrasound Med 2003; 22(6):601–4.

[18] Reinhold C, Tafazoli F, Wang L. Imaging features of adenomyosis. Hum Reprod Update 1998;4(4): 337–49.

[19] Reinhold C, et al. Uterine adenomyosis: endovaginal US and MR imaging features with histopathologic correlation. Radiographics 1999;19: S147–60.

[20] Andreotti RF, Fleischer AC. The sonographic diagnosis of adenomyosis. Ultrasound Q 2005; 21(3):167–70.

[21] Bazot M, et al. Ultrasonography compared with magnetic resonance imaging for the diagnosis of adenomyosis: correlation with histopathology. Hum Reprod 2001;16(11):2427–33.

[22] Bromley B, Shipp TD, Benacerraf B. Adenomyosis: sonographic findings and diagnostic accuracy. J Ultrasound Med 2000;19(8):529–34 [quiz: 535–6].

[23] Atri M, et al. Adenomyosis: US features with histologic correlation in an in-vitro study. Radiology 2000;215(3):783–90.

[24] Ascher SM, et al. Adenomyosis: prospective comparison of MR imaging and transvaginal sonography. Radiology 1994;190(3):803–6.

[25] Reinhold C, et al. Diffuse uterine adenomyosis: morphologic criteria and diagnostic accuracy of endovaginal sonography. Radiology 1995;197(3): 609–14.

[26] Tamai K, et al. MR imaging findings of adenomyosis: correlation with histopathologic features and diagnostic pitfalls. Radiographics 2005;25(1): 21–40.

[27] Hulka CA, et al. Sonographic findings in patients with adenomyosis: can sonography assist in predicting extent of disease? AJR Am J Roentgenol 2002;179(2):379–83.

[28] Chiang CH, et al. Tumor vascular pattern and blood flow impedance in the differential diagnosis of leiomyoma and adenomyosis by color Doppler sonography. J Assist Reprod Genet 1999;16(5):268–75.

[29] Prieto A, et al. Uterine lipoleiomyomas: US and CT findings. Abdom Imaging 2000;25(6): 655–7.

[30] Leibsohn S, et al. Leiomyosarcoma in a series of hysterectomies performed for presumed uterine leiomyomas. Am J Obstet Gynecol 1990;162(4): 968–74 [discussion: 974–6].

[31] Aviram R, et al. Uterine sarcomas versus leiomyomas: gray-scale and Doppler sonographic findings. J Clin Ultrasound 2005;33(1): 10–3.

[32] Hata K, et al. Uterine sarcoma: can it be differentiated from uterine leiomyoma with Doppler ultrasonography? A preliminary report. Ultrasound Obstet Gynecol 1997;9(2):101–4.

[33] Kinkel K. Pitfalls in staging uterine neoplasm with imaging: a review. Abdom Imaging 2006; 31(2):164–73.

[34] Fong K, et al. Transvaginal US and hysterosonography in postmenopausal women with breast cancer receiving tamoxifen: correlation with hysteroscopy and pathologic study. Radiographics 2003;23(1):137–50 [discussion: 151–5].

[35] O'Brien P, et al. Uterine arteriovenous malformations: from diagnosis to treatment. J Ultrasound Med 2006;25(11):1387–92 [quiz: 1394–5].

[36] Murase E, et al. Uterine leiomyomas: histopathologic features, MR imaging findings, differential diagnosis, and treatment. Radiographics 1999; 19(5):1179–97.

[37] Madan R. The bridging vascular sign. Radiology 2006;238(1):371–2.

[38] Kim JC, Kim SS, Park JY. "Bridging vascular sign" in the MR diagnosis of exophytic uterine leiomyoma. J Comput Assist Tomogr 2000;24(1):57–60.

[39] Kim SH, Sim JS, Seong CK. Interface vessels on color/power Doppler US and MRI: a clue to differentiate subserosal uterine myomas from extrauterine tumors. J Comput Assist Tomogr 2001; 25(1):36–42.

[40] Kroencke TJ, et al. Uterine fibroids: contrast-enhanced MR angiography to predict ovarian artery supply—initial experience. Radiology 2006; 241(1):181–9.

[41] Phelan JP. Myomas and pregnancy. Obstet Gynecol Clin North Am 1995;22(4):801–5.

[42] Parker WH, Fu YS, Berek JS. Uterine sarcoma in patients operated on for presumed leiomyoma and rapidly growing leiomyoma. Obstet Gynecol 1994;83(3):414–8.

[43] Oguchi O, et al. Prediction of histopathologic features and proliferative activity of uterine leiomyoma by magnetic resonance imaging prior to GnRH analogue therapy: correlation between T2-weighted images and effect of GnRH analogue. J Obstet Gynaecol 1995;21(2):107–17.

[44] Takahashi K, et al. Value of magnetic resonance imaging in predicting efficacy of GnRH analogue treatment for uterine leiomyoma. Hum Reprod 2001;16(9):1989–94.

[45] Deligdisch L, Hirschmann S, Altchek A. Pathologic changes in gonadotropin releasing hormone agonist analogue treated uterine leiomyomata. Fertil Steril 1997;67(5):837–41.

[46] Jha RC, et al. Symptomatic fibroleiomyomata: MR imaging of the uterus before and after uterine arterial embolization. Radiology 2000; 217(1):228–35.

[47] Katsumori T, Akazawa K, Mihara T. Uterine artery embolization for pedunculated subserosal fibroids. AJR Am J Roentgenol 2005;184(2): 399–402.

[48] Nikolaidis P, et al. Incidence of nonviable leiomyomas on contrast material-enhanced pelvic MR imaging in patients referred for uterine artery embolization. J Vasc Interv Radiol 2005;16(11): 1465–71.

[49] Shimada K, et al. Differentiation between completely hyalinized uterine leiomyomas and ordinary leiomyomas: three-phase dynamic magnetic resonance imaging (MRI) vs. diffusion-weighted MRI with very small b-factors. J Magn Reson Imaging 2004;20(1):97–104.

[50] Reinhold C, et al. Diffuse adenomyosis: comparison of endovaginal US and MR imaging with histopathologic correlation. Radiology 1996; 199(1):151–8.

[51] Brown HK, et al. Uterine junctional zone: correlation between histologic findings and MR imaging. Radiology 1991;179(2):409–13.

[52] Dueholm M, et al. Magnetic resonance imaging and transvaginal ultrasonography for the diagnosis of adenomyosis. Fertil Steril 2001;76(3):588–94.

[53] Jeng CJ, et al. Laparoscopy-guided myometrial biopsy in the definite diagnosis of diffuse adenomyosis. Hum Reprod 2007;22(7):2016–9.

[54] Kim MD, et al. Long-term results of uterine artery embolization for symptomatic adenomyosis. AJR Am J Roentgenol 2007;188(1):176–81.

[55] Pelage JP, et al. Uterine fibroid vascularization and clinical relevance to uterine fibroid embolization. Radiographics 2005;25(Suppl 1):S99–117.

ELSEVIER
SAUNDERS

ULTRASOUND
CLINICS

Ultrasound Clin 2 (2007) 297–309

Ultrasound of Pelvic Inflammatory Disease

Mindy M. Horrow, MD, FACR, FAIUM[a,b],
Shuchi K. Rodgers, MD[a,*], Shabbir Naqvi, MD[a]

Pelvic inflammatory disease (PID) is an infection of the upper genital tract caused by sexually transmitted disease (STD). In addition to the care required during an acute infection, the sequelae of infertility, ectopic pregnancy, and chronic pelvic pain significantly impact the health care system. Data from 1990 show an estimated cost for care of patients with PID at $4.24 billion annually, with 200,000 hospitalized cases and 1,277,700 outpatient cases. From 1984 to 1990, hospitalizations for PID decreased 25%, with only a slight rise in outpatient visits [1]. More recent estimates from the Centers for Disease Control and Prevention approximate 780,000 new cases of acute PID annually [2]. Although it is unclear if this is a true decrease, or just a result of more outpatient care for patients who have PID, most researchers estimate that there is a significant cohort with unrecognized PID. A study in 2004 found the prevalence of chlamydial infection in young adults in the United States was 4.19%. Women, and in particular black women, had higher rates of 4.74 and 13.95%, respectively [3]. The cost of PID to the health care system stems more from the major chronic complications than the cost of treating the acute infection. Chronic complications include infertility, ectopic pregnancy, and chronic pelvic pain. A recent study found the average per-person lifetime cost of PID ranges from $1060 to $3180 [4]. Risk factors for PID are related to exposure to STDs and include earlier age at first sexual intercourse, multiple partners, history of prior STD, and use of vaginal douche [5]. There is also increased risk from an intra-uterine device (IUD), but this is limited to the first few weeks after insertion[1] [6].

Clinical findings

Most cases of PID are caused by *Chlamydia trachomatis* or *Neisseria gonorrhoeae*. Co-infections of these organisms and other bacteria, including: *Streptococcus* species, *Escherichia coli*, *Haemophilus influenza*, *Bacteroides* species, *Peptostreptococcus* and *Peptococcus* are common. Normally, the major barrier to the assent of both normal vaginal flora and pathogens

[a] Department of Radiology, Albert Einstein Medical Center, 5501 Old York Road, Philadelphia, PA 19141-3098, USA
[b] Jefferson Medical College, Thomas Jefferson University, 1025 Walnut Street, Philadelphia, PA 19107, USA
* Corresponding author. Department of Radiology, Albert Einstein Medical Center, 5501 Old York Road, Philadelphia, PA 19141-3098.
E-mail address: rodgerss@einstein.edu (S.K. Rodgers).
[1] The text of this article is adapted from Horrow MM. Ultrasound of pelvic inflammatory disease. Ultrasound Quarterly 2004;20:171–9; with permission.

1556-858X/07/$ – see front matter © 2007 Elsevier Inc. All rights reserved.
ultrasound.theclinics.com

doi:10.1016/j.cult.2007.08.008

is the endocervical canal and its mucus plug. The infectious bacteria damage the endocervical canal, permitting organisms to ascend into the uterus. Other factors may facilitate the spread of disease. Cervical ectopy (extension of endocervical columnar epithelium outward beyond the cervix) produces a larger area that is susceptible to infection. Cervical ectopy occurs more commonly in teenagers, who also represent the age group with the highest incidence of PID. Cervical mucus changes normally during the menstrual cycle, making the cervix more vulnerable to infection at midcycle, when estrogen levels are high and progesterone is relatively low. After ovulation, the mucus becomes more viscous and less penetrable by both sperm and bacteria. Bacteria also may gain easier access to the uterus when the mucus plug is expelled at menstruation [7]. Less frequently, PID occurs as a secondary infection from adjacent processes (ie, appendiceal, diverticular, postsurgical abscesses, or puerperal, and postdilatation and curettage [D & C] complications). Hematogenous spread is rare, but can occur from tuberculosis.

Primary prevention of PID consists of avoiding exposure to STDs. Secondary prevention involves keeping the lower genital infection from ascending into the uterus. This combines disease detection, treatment, and partner notification. Tertiary prevention, which involves preventing an upper genital tract infection from leading to tubal dysfunction and/or obstruction, has been generally disappointing [8].

The initial diagnosis of PID, which is based upon a combination of symptoms, pelvic examination, and laboratory studies, is often incorrect. Molander and colleagues [9] confirmed PID by laparoscopy in only 67% of women who had clinically suspected PID. Laparoscopy, however, is not suitable for a screening procedure. Initially, transabdominal sonography, and now transvaginal sonography with Doppler have been used in the diagnosis of PID.

Ultrasound findings

Despite the widespread use of sonography in the diagnosis and management of patients with pelvic inflammatory disease, there are no large studies evaluating its sensitivity and specificity or overall usefulness [10–12]. Nonetheless, it is a frequently ordered study in patients who have unexplained, acute pelvic pain or in patients with classic symptoms of PID in whom an adequate clinical examination cannot be performed. If demonstration of a pyosalpinx or tubo–ovarian abscess will result in hospitalization, surgery, or follow-up imaging to evaluate nonoperative management, then initial sonography is indicated. In addition, many patients are examined initially by generalists who may feel more confident relying on imaging studies. CT is ordered with increasing frequency to rule out alternative diagnoses such as appendicitis and diverticulitis. Thus, there are more patients in whom CT is the first study to suggest the diagnosis of PID. Though CT is very sensitive for the detection of pelvic abnormalities, it may not be as specific, particularly in differentiating an ovarian from a tubal process, and ultrasound often is obtained after an abnormal CT study to clarify the pathological process and guide management.

As one reviews the imaging literature of the last 20 years, it is clear that the sensitivity and specificity of sonography for PID depends upon the findings one considers to be indicators of PID and the quality of the equipment and the sonographer. Transabdominal imaging is suitable for determining overall

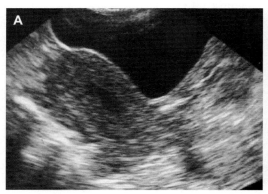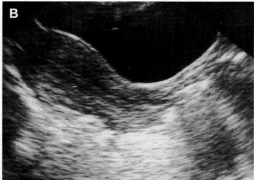

Fig. 1. *(A)* Longitudinal, transabdominal image of the uterus at the time of presentation demonstrates an anteverted, anteflexed uterus with an indistinct endometrial stripe and indistinct margins. *(B)* Re-examination 3 days later after treatment shows a distinct endometrial stripe and uterine margins. (*From* Horrow MM. Ultrasound of pelvic inflammatory disease. Ultrasound Quarterly 2004;20:171–9; with permission.)

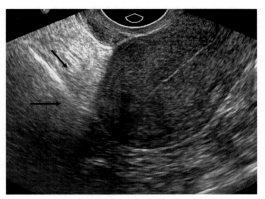

Fig. 2. Sagittal, transvaginal view of the uterus demonstrates prominent echogenic fat *(arrows)* adjacent to the anterior, superior aspect of the uterine fundus.

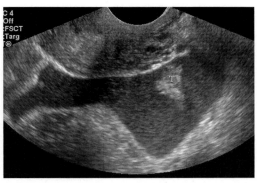

Fig. 4. Transverse, transvaginal view demonstrating complex fluid with low level echoes within the cul de sac from a ruptured hemorrhagic ovarian cyst. The fimbriated portion of a normal fallopian tube (T) is visualized also.

extent of disease. Transvaginal sonography with color or power Doppler, however, has significantly improved the ability to detect subtle abnormalities such as slightly swollen fallopian tubes and to distinguish whether the ovary is involved in an abscess [13]. In addition, many patients who have acute PID cannot tolerate an adequately filled urinary bladder; therefore transabdominal sonography is suboptimal [14]. Papers describing the findings of PID in the pretransvaginal era are therefore of limited use.

In medical imaging, the ability to make the correct diagnosis depends upon knowledge of the possible manifestations of the disease and correlation with the clinical findings. Transvaginal imaging is suited uniquely in both these regards for diagnosing PID. The higher frequency transvaginal probes allow one to observe the more subtle changes of salpingitis and oophoritis. Furthermore, the act of transvaginal imaging itself permits the

sonographer to correlate the patient's symptoms with the imaging findings, by eliciting focal tenderness upon examination of the affected fallopian tubes and ovaries. This is particularly valuable when the imaging findings are subtle.

Acute pelvic inflammatory disease

In a patient without an abscess or pyosalpinx, the manifestations of PID are often subtle and sometimes nonspecific. Mild enlargement or indistinctness of the uterus can be very difficult to appreciate and often only confirmed if a follow-up examination is performed (Fig. 1). If the patient has some fat in the pelvis, inflammatory changes will be manifest as increased echogenicity and prominence of this fat (Fig. 2). It is the authors' experience that subtle changes in uterine size and of the adjacent fat are

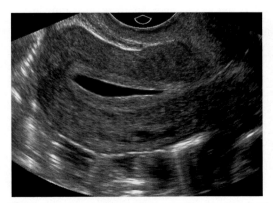

Fig. 3. Sagittal, transvaginal view demonstrates fluid in the endometrial canal consistent with but not specific for endometritis in this patient with pelvic inflammatory disease.

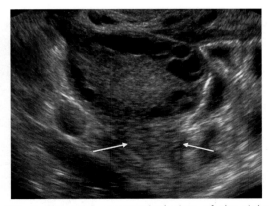

Fig. 5. Transverse, transvaginal view of the right adnexa in a patient with pelvic inflammatory disease demonstrates an enlarged right ovary (volume 23 cc) with multiple tiny peripheral cysts. There is also an adjacent thickened fallopian tube *(arrows)*.

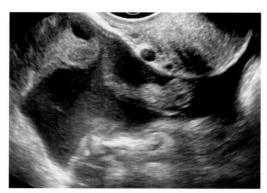

Fig. 6. Transverse, transvaginal image demonstrates a normal fallopian tube outlined by fluid from a ruptured hemorrhagic cyst.

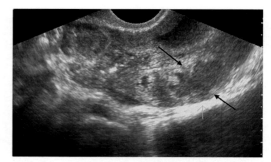

Fig. 8. Transverse, transvaginal view of a fallopian tube *(arrows)* with a thick, echogenic wall, containing complex fluid, representing a pyosalpinx.

appreciated better transabdominally because of the wider field of view. Both fluid in the endometrium and fluid in the cul de sac, common findings in PID, can be found in normal patients and those with alternative diagnoses (Figs. 3 and 4). In addition, some patients who have PID may have little or no free fluid [11]. Nonetheless, the presence of even small amounts of complex pelvic fluid is worrisome for free pus. Careful attention to gain control settings is necessary to visualize internal echoes.

Two groups have reported the finding of enlarged ovaries with increased numbers of small cysts, a so-called polycystic ovary appearance, to correlate with PID (Fig. 5). Cacciatore and colleagues [12] and Golden and colleagues [15] both found larger-than-normal ovarian volumes in their patients who had PID proven by endometrial biopsy or laparoscopy. These authors have found increased ovarian volume to be a useful sign of PID, having documented decreasing volumes on follow-up examinations. A reasonable explanation for this reactive polycystic change is that the inflammation increases ovarian volume by thickening the stroma

and increasing the number and size of cysts. The margins of the ovaries also may become indistinct in PID.

Sonographic findings of the fallopian tubes are the most striking and specific landmarks of PID. Normal fallopian tubes are difficult to visualize on routine transvaginal sonography, unless outlined by fluid (Fig. 6). The normal fallopian tube is approximately 10 cm long and runs along the superior margin of the broad ligament. It can be divided into four segments from the proximal uterine end to the distal fimbriated end as follows: interstitial, isthmic, ampullary, and infundibular. The fimbriated portion of the infundibular segment attaches to the ovary and is open to the peritoneal cavity [16]. The diameter of the tube typically varies between 1 and 4 mm, and in the authors' experience is thickest in the infundibular segment.

When inflamed, the fallopian tube swells, and the walls and endosalpingeal folds thicken, allowing visualization with ultrasound (Fig. 7). This initial stage corresponds to salpingitis, a thickened fallopian tube without intraluminal pus. On ultrasound, it can appear as an indistinct, elongated, noncystic mass in close proximity to the

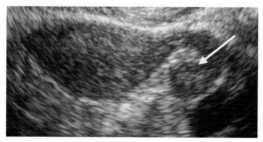

Fig. 7. Transverse view of the pelvis with thickened left fallopian tube *(arrow),* not filled with fluid. *(From* Horrow MM. Ultrasound of Pelvic Inflammatory Disease. Ultrasound Quarterly 2004;20:171–9; with permission.)

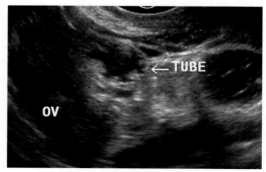

Fig. 9. Transverse, transvaginal view of a slightly dilated, fluid-filled fallopian tube with thickened endosalpingeal folds demonstrating the cog wheel sign.

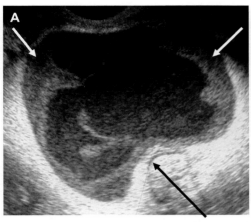
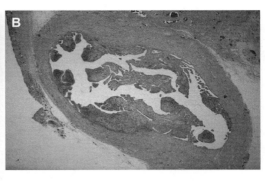

Fig. 10. (A) Cross section of significantly dilated tube *(arrows)* containing echogenic fluid that outlines thickened endosalpingeal folds, demonstrating the cog wheel sign. (B) Photomicrograph of same tube in cross section with thickened folds projecting into a dilated lumen. (*From* Horrow MM. Ultrasound of pelvic inflammatory disease. Ultrasound Quarterly 2004;20:171–9; with permission.)

ovary, but separated from it. The endosalpingeal folds are difficult to discern given the lack of intraluminal fluid as a contrast. The pus may flow freely from the tube into the peritoneum, preventing distention and detection of a thickened tubal wall.

As the lumen occludes distally, the fallopian tube distends and fills with complex fluid, resulting in a pyosalpinx. Various appearances result, as described by Timor-Tritsh and colleagues [17]. The tube becomes ovoid or pear-shaped, filling with fluid that may be anechoic or echogenic, with layers. The wall becomes thickened, greater than or equal to 5 mm (Fig. 8), and incomplete septi are common as the tube folds back upon itself. If the distended tube is viewed in cross section, it may demonstrate the cog wheel sign (Figs. 9 and 10A), because of the thickened endosalpingeal folds (Fig. 10B) [17]. Typically the swollen fallopian tubes extend posteriorly into the cul de sac, rather than extending superiorly and anterior to the uterus as large ovarian tumors tend to do. Fluid debris levels often are visualized in the dilated tubes (Fig. 11), and very rarely gas/fluid levels or bubbles of gas (Fig. 12).

As the disease progresses, the ovary can become involved. Theoretically, a defect in the ovary at the time of ovulation allows bacteria to enter, spreading the infection. When the ovary adheres to the tube, but remains visualized, this indicates a tubo–ovarian complex (Fig. 13). A tubo–ovarian abscess is the result of a complete breakdown of ovarian and tubal architecture such that separate structures no longer are identified (Fig. 14). Without treatment, a tubo–ovarian abscess can rupture, resulting in peritonitis and multiple intra-abdominal abscesses (Fig. 15). If the contralateral side was

not affected initially, the disease may spread there secondarily. When both tubes are inflamed and occluded, the entire complex typically takes on a U shape as it fills the cul de sac, extending from one adnexal region to the other. The lateral and posterior borders of the uterus become obscured, and individual tubes and ovaries cannot be distinguished.

Color and power Doppler may show increased flow (hyperemia) in the walls and incomplete septi of the inflamed tubes (Fig. 16). In the acute phase of the infection, the mean resistive and pulsatility indices may be low, measuring 0.5 (standard deviation [SD] = 0.05) and 0.79 (SD = 0.12). With treatment, these values increased to 0.63 and 1.17, respectively [18]. Some authors have shown that

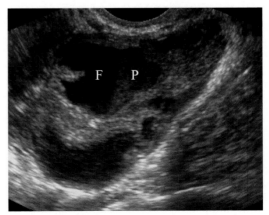

Fig. 11. Oblique, transvaginal view of a dilated right fallopian tube containing a fluid–pus level.

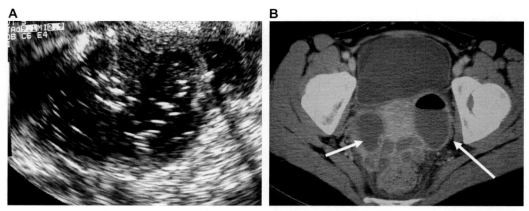

Fig. 12. (A) Dilated left fallopian tube filled with fluid and multiple bright echogenic foci representing bubbles of gas. (B) CT image through the pelvis in the same patient shows dilated tubes (arrows) filling the cul de sac. The left tube contains a gas/fluid level. (From Horrow MM. Ultrasound of pelvic inflammatory disease. Ultrasound Quarterly 2004;20:171–9; with permission.)

patients who responded to conservative, medical treatment tended to have a higher resistive index (.6 ± .15) than those who required surgery (.52 ± .08), although there was significant overlap between the two groups [19]. It is the authors' experience that color Doppler imaging can be useful to differentiate PID from tumors or masses, but specific resistive and pulsatility indices are not helpful. Decreased flow on follow-up imaging may be useful to assess for response to therapy.

Chronic pelvic inflammatory disease

Chronic PID typically results in a hydrosalpinx from accumulation of fluid caused by occlusion of the tube distally or at both ends. Other causes of hydrosalpinx, however, include tubal ligation,

following hysterectomy if the fallopian tubes are left in to protect the vascular supply to the ovary, and primary or secondary tumors of the fallopian tubes [16]. Several specific ultrasound findings can help distinguish a hydrosalpinx from other cystic adnexal lesions. A hydrosalpinx tends to be anechoic, more tubular, and often demonstrates the incomplete septa sign (Fig. 17). The tubal wall is thin, less than 5 mm, and in cross section demonstrates the beads-on-a-string sign (Fig. 18) [17]. These beads are 2 to 3 mm hyperechoic nodules projecting from the wall, representing remnants of the endosalpingeal folds. If color flow is detected in a hydrosalpinx, it tends to be less exuberant than in acute PID. Molander and colleagues [9] found a higher pulsatility index in patients who had a chronic hydrosalpinx (1.5 ± .1) than with

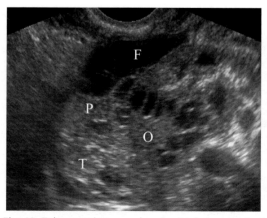

Fig. 13. Tubo–ovarian complex. Sagittal, transvaginal image of the left adnexa demonstrates an ovary (O) with ill-defined borders, surrounded by a thickened fallopian tube (T) containing fluid (F) and pus (P).

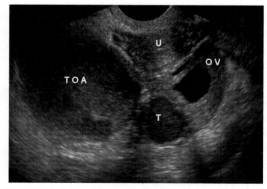

Fig. 14. Transverse, transvaginal image of the pelvis demonstrates a right tubo–ovarian abscess (TOA) and a left tubo–ovarian complex consisting of a pyosalpinx (T) and the adjacent left ovary (OV).

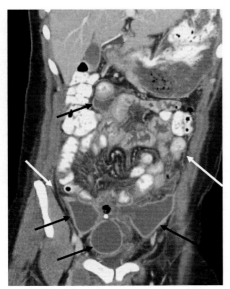

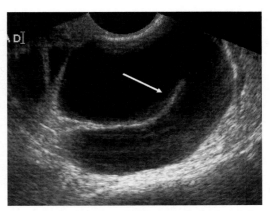

Fig. 17. Sagittal, transvaginal image of a hydrosalpinx, demonstrating an incomplete septum *(arrow)*.

Fig. 15. Coronal enhanced CT scan in a different patient demonstrating peritoneal inflammation *(white arrows)* and multiple abscesses *(black arrows)* from a ruptured tubo–ovarian abscess.

acute PID (.84 ± .04). Occasional patients with prior PID may demonstrate a peritoneal inclusion cyst. This diagnosis is made when the ovary is surrounded by a loculated fluid collection with thin septations [20]. A peritoneal inclusion cyst forms

when fluid from a ruptured ovarian cyst is trapped around the ovary by adhesions (Fig. 19).

Sonographic changes can occur fairly rapidly after treatment of PID. Minor findings such as complex fluid and inflammation in the surrounding fat can resolve in a few days. A pyosalpinx can change to a hydrosalpinx and possibly resolve over a few weeks to several months. Interestingly, Taipale and colleagues [21] found that 9 of 55 patients who had clinical PID and an initial, normal sonogram developed a hydrosalpinx with time. If a pyosalpinx does not resolve or develops into

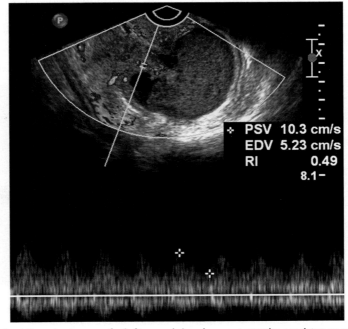

Fig. 16. Color and pulsed Doppler image of a left pyosalpinx demonstrates low resistance arterial flow (RI = .49).

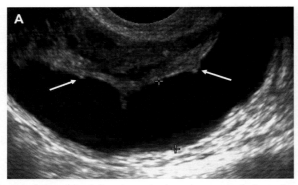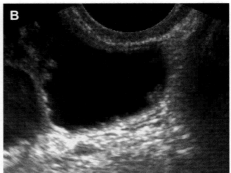

Fig. 18. (A) Hydrosalpinx. Lengthwise, transvaginal view of a dilated, fluid-filled fallopian tube demonstrating residual endosalpingeal folds *(arrows)*. (B) Cross section of the same tube shows the beads on a string sign.

a hydrosalpinx, it probably signifies an incompletely treated infection.

Related findings and differential diagnosis

Patients who have severe PID can develop a reactive ileus (Fig. 20), which can be visualized during sonographic evaluation of the pelvis. Perihepatitis associated with PID is known as Fitz-Hugh-Curtis Syndrome, which occurs in 3% to 10% of patients who have PID [22]. The acute right upper quadrant pain often overshadows the pelvic pain because of acute salpingitis. Inflammatory exudates in the pouch of Douglas spread along the peritoneal surface to the anterior surface of the liver by means of the paracolic gutter (Fig. 21). Often alternative diagnoses such as cholecystitis are considered first, and imaging of the right upper quadrant may be requested. Shoenfeld and colleagues [23] found thickening of the right anterior extrarenal fascia

on ultrasound in nine patients. Scattered cases of Fitz-Hugh-Curtis syndrome on CT have demonstrated increased enhancement of the peritoneal surface of the anterior aspect of the liver, gallbladder wall thickening, and a transient hepatic attenuation difference [24,25].

Though the combination of sonographic and clinical findings is often quite specific for PID, there are several other common diagnoses in the differential diagnosis. The most common alternative diagnoses with findings which simulate PID by the presence of an indistinct uterus and complex pelvic fluid, are ruptured hemorrhagic cyst and endometrioma. Perforated appendicitis and ruptured tubo-ovarian abscess may present with indistinguishable findings of peritonitis and intra-abdominal abscesses. Other tubular structures in the pelvis which bear a resemblance to dilated fallopian tubes but should be distinguishable from them include

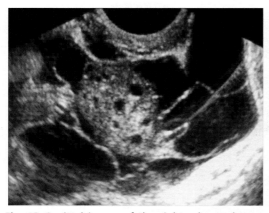

Fig. 19. Sagittal image of the right adnexa demonstrating loculated fluid with thin septations, surrounding the right ovary compatible with a peritoneal inclusion cyst. The patient has a history of pelvic inflammatory disease.

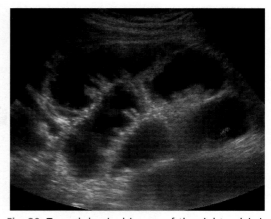

Fig. 20. Transabdominal image of the right pelvis in a patient with pelvic inflammatory disease demonstrates dilated loops of small bowel without peristalsis, compatible with a reactive ileus.

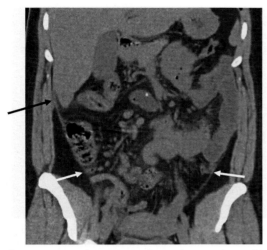

Fig. 21. Fitz-Hugh-Curtis syndrome in a patient with pelvic inflammatory disease. Coronal unenhanced CT image demonstrates peritoneal inflammation *(white arrows)* extending to the inferior liver capsule *(black arrow)*. The patient presented with right upper quadrant pain.

an inflamed appendix (Fig. 22), a hydroureter, prominent pelvic veins (Fig. 23), and varices.

Septic ovarian vein or pelvic vein thrombophlebitis may present with a similar clinical picture as PID. However, it most commonly occurs postpartum, but can be associated with pelvic trauma, PID, or recent pelvic surgery. In the majority of cases, it occurs on the right side, and during the first week postpartum. On sonography, a tubular anechoic or hypoechoic structure is identified, extending superiorly from the adnexa, with absence of flow on Doppler imaging (Fig. 24) [26].

A hydrosalpinx can mimic a cystic ovarian mass. This occurs when a significantly scarred hydrosalpinx has multiple septa without connecting compartments. Conversely, cystic ovarian tumors seldom have incomplete septa. Large para-tubal or para-ovarian cysts can also appear similar to a hydrosalpinx. For example, a hydatid of Morgagni is a benign cystic structure arising from a müllerian duct vestige adjacent to the fimbrial end of the fallopian tube (Fig. 25). Identification of the ovary separate from the hydrosalpinx allows differentiation from an ovarian mass. MRI or CT may aid in difficult cases.

Torsion of the fallopian tube is a rare condition that can occur with PID or other pre-disposing conditions. These include hydrosalpinx, tubal tortuosity, tubal ligation, tumor, or extrinsic causes such as a paratubal mass, adjacent adhesions, or enlargement of the uterus compressing the tube. The clinical presentation is similar to ovarian torsion. Sonography typically shows a thick-walled distended fallopian tube, which may contain hemorrhage. Differentiation of acute PID with tubal pus from tubal torsion with hematosalpinx may be difficult. Since tubal blood supply is from both ovarian and uterine vessels, the presence of flow on color Doppler does not exclude the diagnosis. Ultimately, the prospective diagnosis of tubal torsion is very difficult and is most often made pathologically [16,27].

Other imaging: CT

When significant sonographic findings are detected in the pelvis, sonography should be extended into the abdomen. Complex pelvic fluid may ascend into the flanks and Morison's pouch. Hydroureteronephrosis is not uncommon. Patients with nausea

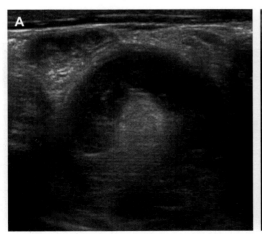
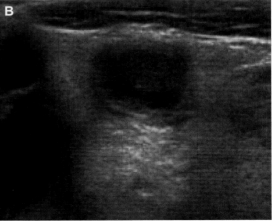

Fig. 22. (A) Transabdominal view of the right adnexa demonstrates a tubular, blind ending structure with low-level internal echoes. Patient had surgically proven appendicitis. *(B)* Transverse view of the same dilated appendix with surrounding echogenic fat consistent with inflammation.

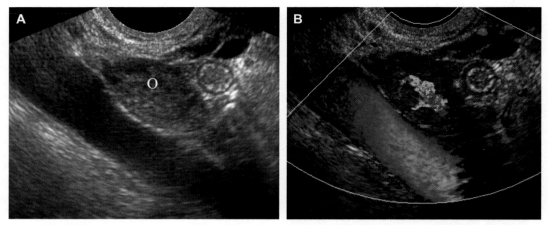

Fig. 23. (A) Sagittal, transvaginal view of the right adnexa demonstrates a tubular structure adjacent to the right ovary (O). *(B)* Corresponding color Doppler image demonstrates that the tubular structure represents a prominent iliac vein.

and vomiting often demonstrate dilated loops of small bowel with minimal peristalsis, indicative of an ileus.

While ultrasound remains the imaging modality of choice in cases of suspected PID, if the symptoms are more generalized and non-specific, CT is often ordered first. CT should be performed with both oral and intravenous contrast. While many of the classic sonographic findings including enlarged ovaries, dilated tubes and free-fluid are equally well seen on CT, the mild inflammatory changes of PID may be better appreciated on CT than ultrasound. Mild pelvic edema causes thickening of the utero–sacral ligaments and haziness of pelvic fat [28]. Periovarian stranding and enhancement of the peritoneum, endometrium and endocervical canal are well visualized with CT (Figs. 26 and 27).

CT is also beneficial in detecting involvement of adjacent structures such as: small and/or large bowel ileus or obstruction, ureteral obstruction, secondary inflammation of the appendix and inflammation of the greater omentum. The extent of a ruptured tubo-ovarian abscess is better appreciated with CT. In contrast to ultrasound however, it is more difficult to differentiate a pyosalpinx from a tubo-ovarian complex or abscess by CT. Similarly mildly dilated tubes may go unrecognized on CT. A subgroup of patients with an intra-uterine contraceptive device in place may develop a particular type of subacute or indolent form of PID. They are prone to infection with Actinomyces israelii, leading to a more chronic, suppurative infection which may simulate a neoplasm with carcinomatosis on CT [29].

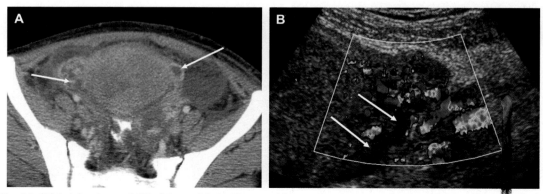

Fig. 24. (A) Axial enhanced CT of the pelvis in 13-year-old recently postpartum patient shows bilateral tubular low density structures with enhancing walls, compatible with thrombosed, septic pelvic veins. *(B)* Corresponding transverse color Doppler image shows hypoechoic thrombus in a left pelvic vein.

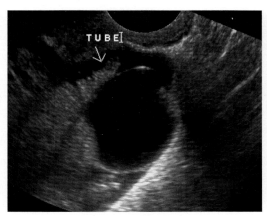

Fig. 25. Transverse, transvaginal view of the left adnexa demonstrates a paratubal cyst (Hydatid of Morgagni) arising from the fimbriated portion of the left fallopian tube.

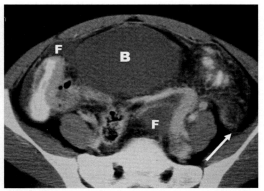

Fig. 27. CT scan through superior aspect of pelvis shows distended bladder (B) and inflammation of peritoneal fat *(arrow)*. The anterior peritoneum is thickened and enhancing, and small collections of fluid are present (F). (*From* Horrow MM. Ultrasound of pelvic inflammatory disease. Ultrasound Quarterly 2004;20:171–9; with permission.)

Other imaging: MRI

Scattered reports of MR imaging for PID show findings similar to CT. Pelvic inflammation appears as ill-defined hyperintense areas on fat-suppressed T2 weighted images and marked enhancement on gadolinium-enhanced fat-suppressed T1-weighted images. Contents of a pyosalpinx or abscess are slightly hyperintense on T1-weighted images and slightly hypointense on T2-weighted images relative to urine due to hemorrhage or debris. The superior tissue contrast and multiplanar capability of MRI is occasionally useful in problem solving difficult

ultrasound cases (Fig. 28). For example, MRI can distinguish hematosalpinx from pyosalpinx, both of which can look similar on ultrasound.

In a study comparing ultrasound and MRI in a group of 21 patients with PID proven at laparoscopy, sensitivity and specificity for PID was 95% and 89% by MRI and 81% and 78% for ultrasound [30]. The authors felt that MRI was better than ultrasound for distinguishing other causes of cystic adnexal masses when a dilated tube was not present. Also, MRI was more sensitive for small amounts of fluid throughout the pelvis. Nonetheless, the significantly lower cost and easier availability of ultrasound makes it the initial imaging study of choice, with MRI used selectively for problem solving in complex or equivocal cases.

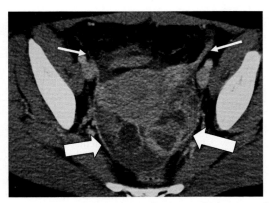

Fig. 26. CT scan through pelvis shows thickening of the broad ligaments *(thin arrows)* and thickening and enhancement of the peritoneum in the cul de sac *(thick arrows)*. The cul de sac contains fluid and dilated fallopian tubes. (*From* Horrow MM. Ultrasound of pelvic inflammatory disease. Ultrasound Quarterly 2004;20:171–9; with permission.)

Summary

Though the true sensitivity and specificity of ultrasound for PID are unknown, this study is frequently ordered. Awareness of the subtle findings of PID, particularly those that distinguish a dilated fallopian tube from other cystic adnexal masses ("incomplete septa," "cog wheel," and "beads-on-a-string" signs) will allow the interpreter to be more accurate. Transvaginal scanning allows one to correlate imaging findings with symptoms. As CT is used with increasing frequency, imagers must be able to appreciate the findings of PID on this modality and when to correlate with sonography.

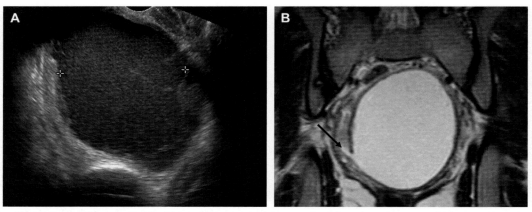

Fig. 28. (A) Transverse, transvaginal image demonstrating a cystic right adnexal mass with fine, uniform low-level echoes and peripheral echogenic mural nodule, highly suggestive of an endometrioma. (B) Coronal T2-weighted MR image shows lumen of the same cystic mass continuous with the adjacent fallopian tube (arrow), indicating that it is tubal in origin. Surgical pathology proved this structure to be a pyosalpinx.

References

[1] Washington AE, Katz P. Cost of and payment source for pelvic inflammatory disease: trends and projections, 1983 through 2000. JAMA 1991;266:2565–9.

[2] Rein DB, Kassler WJ, Irwin KL, et al. Direct medical cost of pelvic inflammatory disease and its sequelae: decreasing but still substantial. Obstet Gynecol 2000;95:397–402.

[3] Miller WC, Ford CA, Morris M, et al. Prevalence of chlamydial and gonococcal infections among young adults in the United States. JAMA 2004; 291:2229–36.

[4] Yeh JM, Hook EW, Goldie SJ. A refined estimate of the average lifetime cost of pelvic inflammatory disease. Sex Transm Dis 2003;30:369–78.

[5] Aral SO, Mosher WD, Cates W Jr. Self-reported pelvic inflammatory disease in the United States, 1988. JAMA 1991;266:2570–3.

[6] Barrett S, Taylor C. A review on pelvic inflammatory disease. Int J STD AIDS 2005;16:715–21.

[7] Rice PA, Schachter J. Pathogenesis of pelvic inflammatory disease: what are the questions? JAMA 1991;266:2587–93.

[8] Washington AE, Cates W, Wasserheit JN. Preventing pelvic inflammatory disease. JAMA 1991;266: 2574–80.

[9] Molander P, Sjoberg J, Paavonen J, et al. Transvaginal power Doppler findings in laparoscopically proven acute pelvic inflammatory disease. Ultrasound Obstet Gynecol 2002;17:233–8.

[10] Patten RM, Vincent LM, Wolner-Hanssen P, et al. Pelvic inflammatory disease: endovaginal sonography with laparoscopic correlation. J Ultrasound Med 1990;9:681–9.

[11] Boardman LA, Peipert JF, Brody JM, et al. Endovaginal sonography for the diagnosis of upper genital tract infection. Obstet and Gynecol 1997;90:54–7.

[12] Cacciatore B, Leminen A, Ingman-Friberg S, et al. Transvaginal sonographic findings in ambulatory patients with suspected pelvic inflammatory disease. Obstet Gynecol 1992;80:912–6.

[13] Bulas DI, Ahlstrom PA, Sivit CJ, et al. Pelvic inflammatory disease in the adolescent: comparison of transabdominal and transvaginal sonographic evaluation. Radiology 1992; 183:435–9.

[14] Bellah RD, Rosenberg HK. Transvaginal ultrasound in a children's hospital: is it worthwhile? Pediatr Radiol 1991;21:570–4.

[15] Golden N, Cohen H, Gennari G, et al. The use of pelvic ultrasonography in the evaluation of adolescents with pelvic inflammatory disease. Am J Dis Child 1987;141:1235–8.

[16] Benjaminov O, Atri M. Sonography of the abnormal fallopian tube. AJR Am J Roentgenol 2004; 183:737–42.

[17] Timor-Tritsch IE, Lerner JP, Monteagudo A, et al. Transvaginal sonographic markers of tubal inflammatory disease. Ultrasound Obstet Gynecol 1998;12:56–66.

[18] Tinkanen H, Kujansuu E. Doppler ultrasound findings in tubo–ovarian infectious complex. J Clin Ultrasound 1993;21:175–7.

[19] Tepper R, Aviram R, Cohen N, et al. Doppler flow characteristics in patients with pelvic inflammatory disease: responders versus nonresponders to therapy. J Clin Ultrasound 1998; 26:247–9.

[20] Horrow MM, Brown KJ. Femscan: multiloculated pelvic cyst. Journal of Women's Imaging 2002;4: 89–90.

[21] Taipale P, Tarjanne H, Ylostalo P. Transvaginal sonography in suspected pelvic inflammatory disease. Ultrasound Obstet Gynecol 1995;6:430–4.

[22] Ignacio E, Hill M. Ultrasound of the acute female pelvis. Ultrasound Q 2003;19:86–98.

[23] Schoenfeld A, Fisch B, Cohen M, et al. Ultrasound findings in perihepatitis associated with pelvic inflammatory disease. J Clin Ultrasound 1992;20:339–42.

[24] Tsubuku M, Hayashi S, Terahara A, et al. Fitz-Hugh-Curtis syndrome: linear contrast enhancement of the surface of the liver on CT. J Comput Assist Tomogr 2002;26:456–8.

[25] Pickhardt PJ, Fleishman MJ, Fisher AJ. Fitz-Hugh-Curtis syndrome: multidetector CT findings of transient hepatic attenuation difference and gallbladder wall thickening. AJR Am J Roentgenol 2003;180:1605–6.

[26] Quane LK, Kidney DD, Cohen AJ. Unusual causes of ovarian vein thrombosis as revealed by CT and Sonography. AJR Am J Roentgenol 1998;171:487–90.

[27] Gross M, Blumstein SL, Chow LC. Isolated fallopian tube torsion: a rare twist on a common theme. AJR Am J Roentgenol 2005;185:1590–2.

[28] Sam JW, Jacobs JE, Birnbaum BA. Spectrum of CT findings in acute pyogenic pelvic inflammatory disease. RadioGraphics 2002;22:1327–34.

[29] Lee I-J, Ha HK, Park CM, et al. Abdominopelvic actinomycosis involving the gastrointestinal tract: CT features. Radiology 2001;220:76–80.

[30] Tukeva TA, Aronen HJ, Karjalainen PT, et al. MR imaging in pelvic inflammatory disease: comparison with laparoscopy and US. Radiology 1999; 210:209–16.

ELSEVIER
SAUNDERS

ULTRASOUND
CLINICS

Ultrasound Clin 2 (2007) 311–325

Imaging of Adnexal Torsion

Leslie M. Scoutt, MD[a],*, Oksana H. Baltarowich, MD[b],
Anna S. Lev-Toaff, MD[c]

- Clinical presentation
- US findings of ovarian torsion
- CT appearance of ovarian torsion

- MR appearance of ovarian torsion
- Summary
- References

Adnexal torsion is estimated to account for approximately 3% of all gynecologic emergencies ranking in frequency behind ectopic pregnancy, ruptured ovarian cyst, pelvic inflammatory disease and appendicitis [1,2]. Prompt diagnosis is essential to prevent ovarian infarction and necrosis. While women with ovarian torsion classically present with sudden onset of severe pelvic pain, many patients present with mild or intermittent symptoms. Hence, the diagnosis may not be considered and patients are often initially evaluated for renal or gastrointestinal pathology as well as other gynecologic causes of lower quadrant pain. While ultrasound (US) is the imaging modality of choice for evaluation of women with suspected gynecologic pathology, a computed tomography (CT) scan is often the first diagnostic imaging test obtained if the presentation is non-specific or if the clinician suspects renal colic or bowel pathology such as appendicitis or diverticulitis. Magnetic resonance imaging (MRI) is considered an important second order imaging technique if US or CT findings are equivocal, although MR is preferred over CT for imaging pregnant women to avoid exposing the fetus to ionizing radiation. Thus, patients with adnexal torsion may be imaged initially with CT or MR and, hence, the

radiologist should be familiar with the appearance of adnexal torsion on these modalities as well as on US. This article reviews the US as well as CT and MR findings of adnexal torsion.

Clinical presentation

Adnexal torsion is caused by twisting of the ovary and/or fallopian tube around its vascular pedicle. Most commonly both the ovary and ipsilateral fallopian tube are torsed together. Adnexal torsion occurs most often on the right [3,4], and is usually unilateral. Hypotheses for the right-sided predominance include decreased space in the left pelvis due to the presence of the sigmoid colon, mobility of the cecum, differences in venous drainage, and increase in the length and/or mobility of the right adnexal supporting structures and vascular pedicle [3]. The degree of torsion is variable ranging from partial (90°) to multiple twists (up to 720°). Initially, venous and/or lymphatic obstruction occurs and the ovary becomes enlarged and edematous. If the torquing of the vascular pedicle is not relieved, arterial flow to the ovary is ultimately impaired resulting in hemorrhagic infarction. The length of time from onset of pain to non-reversible ovarian necrosis is

[a] Department of Diagnostic Radiology, Yale University School of Medicine, 20 York Street, 2-272 WP, New Haven, CT 06504, USA
[b] Department of Radiology, Thomas Jefferson University, 132 S. 10th Street, 796B Main Bldg., Philadelphia, PA 19107-5244, USA
[c] Department of Radiology, Thomas Jefferson University, 132 S. 10th Street, 763L Main Bldg., Philadelphia, PA 19107-5244, USA
* Corresponding author.
E-mail address: leslie.scoutt@yale.edu (L.M. Scoutt).

1556-858X/07/$ – see front matter © 2007 Elsevier Inc. All rights reserved.
ultrasound.theclinics.com

doi:10.1016/j.cult.2007.10.001

reported to be highly variable; likely due to the following factors: 1) wide variation in both the degree and duration of torsion, 2) dual arterial blood supply to the ovary such that some blood flow to the ovary may be maintained despite occlusion of one arterial source, and 3) the fact that ovarian torsion is commonly intermittent. However, in the absence of spontaneous detorsion, surgical intervention to untwist the vascular pedicle is necessary to prevent ovarian necrosis and to preserve ovarian function. In the past, oophorectomy was routinely performed in patients with ovarian torsion due to the perceived risk of pulmonary embolus from gonadal vein thrombosis. Currently, this risk is not felt to be significant [5–7] and if the ovary is felt to be viable on surgical inspection, it is untwisted and oophoropexy is performed. However, the ovarian salvage rate is estimated to be only approximately 10% [1,8]. The most likely explanations for the low ovarian salvage rate following surgical detorsion are delay in diagnosis and difficulty in assessing ovarian viability on surgical inspection as sometimes a necrotic appearing ovary may subsequently prove to be viable [6].

Delay in diagnosis is primarily due to the non-specific clinical presentation of many patients with adnexal torsion. Classically, patients with ovarian torsion present with acute onset of severe, sharp lower quadrant pain which is frequently associated with nausea and vomiting. The pain may radiate to the groin or thigh, and patients may have a mass or rebound tenderness on physical examination. Patients are usually afebrile with a normal white blood cell count. However, a low grade fever or mild leukocytosis may be observed [1,5,6,8–10]. In patients with classic signs and symptoms, the clinical concern for ovarian torsion is very high and work-up proceeds quickly with emergent US examination. However, in many patients the pelvic pain may be much less severe, intermittent, or of several day's duration, and the correct diagnosis may not be initially suspected [1,4,8]. In patients with such non-specific clinical presentation, the differential diagnosis is broad and includes gynecologic as well as renal and gastrointestinal pathology such as ruptured or hemorrhagic ovarian cysts, pelvic inflammatory disease, ectopic pregnancy, renal colic, diverticulitis, appendicitis, colitis, small bowel obstruction and intussusception. One series estimated that the accuracy of clinical diagnosis for ovarian torsion was only 37.8% and that 20% of women with ovarian torsion underwent elective operation with another presumptive diagnosis, most often ruptured ovarian cyst or abscess, due to lack of impressive or specific symptoms [1]. In another series of 87 patients with ovarian torsion, the admitting diagnosis was ovarian torsion in only 47% of patients and only 26 patients underwent surgery within 24 hours [8]. Many authors acknowledge that the diagnosis is more difficult to make during pregnancy, in the postmenopausal patient, or in patients with underlying adnexal masses [7,9,10].

Ovarian torsion occurs most commonly during the reproductive years, likely related to ovulation.

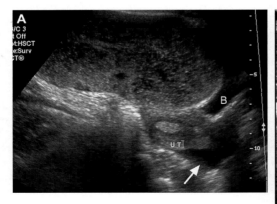
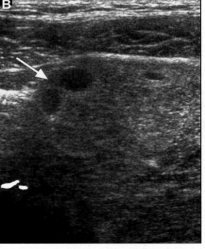

Fig. 1. (*A*) Sagittal greyscale US image demonstrates a large midline solid avascular mass of heterogeneous echotexture superior to the uterus (UT) in child presenting with acute abdominal pain and an abdominal mass on physical exam. Bladder (*B*). Note free fluid in the cul de sac (*arrow*). (*B*) High resolution image obtained with a linear array transducer demonstrates small peripheral cystic spaces (*arrow*) representing displaced follicles, which helped to confirm the diagnosis of ovarian torsion. Central hypoechoic areas are likely due to edema. (*Courtesy* of Dr. T. Robin Goodman, MD, New Haven, CT.)

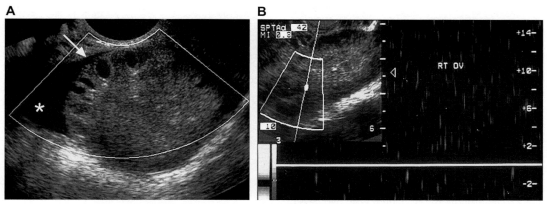

Fig. 2. (*A*) Color Doppler image demonstrates an enlarged avascular right ovary with heterogenous central stroma and several peripherally located follicles (*arrow*) in this 24 year old woman with acute onset of RLQ pain due to ovarian torsion. Note a small amount of adjacent free fluid (*). (*B*) Pulse Doppler interrogation demonstrates no evidence of either arterial or venous blood flow.

However, adnexal torsion has been reported in utero, in neonates, in premenarchal children as well as in postmenopausal women. In the Mayo Clinic series, 27% of patients with proven adnexal torsion were postmenopausal [9]. Chiou and colleagues [10] reported that 24% of the patients with adnexal torsion in their series were postmenopausal. Predisposing risk factors for adnexal torsion include underlying ipsilateral ovarian mass, pregnancy, ovarian hyperstimulation syndrome, prior pelvic surgery and hypermobility of adnexal structures. An underlying mass is found in 50-81% of all cases of adnexal torsion [1,4,10,11]. Underlying pathology is reportedly most common in postmenopausal women and least common in adolescents and children. In one series, an ipsilateral adnexal mass was noted in 86% of postmenopausal women with adnexal torsion [10]. The mass is believed to act as a fulcrum providing mass effect or momentum allowing torsion to occur. Dermoid cysts are the most common underlying lesion with a reported incidence of 20-37% [1,12]. However, the risk of torsion for a dermoid was actually less than for para-ovarian cysts, solid benign tumors or serous cysts in one series [1]. Hibbard [1] has reported that malignant ovarian neoplasms are less likely to undergo torsion (2.4%) in comparison to benign ovarian lesions (11%). Peritumoral adhesions, inflammation, or invasion of local structures may prevent torsion of malignant ovarian neoplasms. Nonetheless, torsion of ovarian malignancies can occur [9,10] with an incidence as high as 15% reported in the Mayo Clinic series although this series had an unusually high number of postmenopausal women [9]. Ovarian size >6 cm is believed to increase the risk of torsion in adults although very large lesions rarely undergo torsion as they are likely stabilized by surrounding pelvic structures.

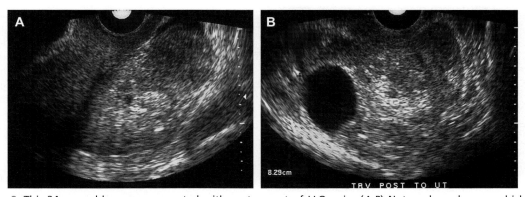

Fig. 3. This 34 year old woman presented with acute onset of LLQ pain. (*A,B*) Note enlarged ovary which is located midline in the cul de sac and demonstrates prominent irregular echogenic areas consistent with hemorrhage. Edematous tissue is more hypoechoic. Note underlying ovarian cyst on image (*B*). The ovary was infarcted at surgical exploration.

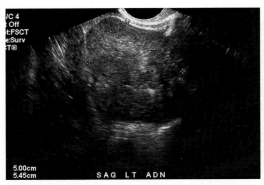

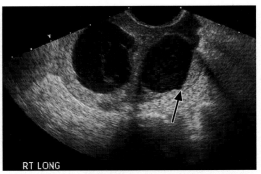

Fig. 4. The left ovary (calipers) is enlarged, heterogenous and amorphous in this patient with two days of pelvic pain due to ovarian torsion.

Fig. 6. In this patient with ovarian torsion the ovary is enlarged with a complex appearance due to the presence of two hemorrhage ovarian cysts. Arrow denotes layering blood.

Up to 12-24% of all cases of ovarian torsion are reported to occur during pregnancy [3,4,7,11,13,14]. Many of these cases (~60%) are associated with ovulation induction and enlarged ovaries in patients with ovarian hyperstimulation syndrome [3,7,11]. As many as 40-48% of patients with ovarian torsion give a history of prior pelvic surgery (most often tubal ligation) and it is hypothesized that post-surgical adhesions provide a fixed structure in the pelvis around which the ovarian pedicle might twist [8,10]. In the study report by Pena and colleagues [3], 29% of patients with ovarian torsion had undergone prior tubal ligation. Hypermobility of the adnexa is believed to be a cause of torsion, particularly in children (see below), and may also be a factor in patients who have undergone tubal ligation.

Adnexal torsion is less common in children than in adults but it is estimated that close to 15% of cases occur in neonates, prepubertal and adolescent girls [1]. The diagnosis should be considered in children who present with either acute or intermittent lower quadrant pain, especially if associated with nausea, vomiting or an adnexal/abdominal mass (**Fig. 1**) [6]. However, as in adults, the clinical presentation can mimic appendicitis, renal colic, pelvic inflammatory disease and ruptured or hemorrhagic ovarian cysts. In neonates and prepubertal girls the enlarged torsed ovary is frequently extra pelvic in location, usually in the abdomen or inguinal canal. Stark reported that in young girls with ovarian torsion, the enlarged ovary was palpated outside of the pelvis in 81% cases whereas the twisted ovary was located within the pelvis in all older or pubertal girls [15]. Many cases of adnexal torsion in children are associated with underlying adnexal pathology, most commonly cystic teratomas or functional ovarian cysts [6,16]. Cystic epithelial neoplasms, solid tumors, and malignant ovarian lesions have a lower incidence of torsion. However, large ovarian lesions are less likely to twist in children than in adults. Warner and colleagues [17] reported that ovarian cysts >5 cm rarely cause ovarian torsion in children. The ovaries are morphologically normal in at least 16-25% of children with ovarian torsion, particularly in younger girls [6,16]. Excessive mobility, tortuosity or elongation of the fallopian tube, vessels, mesosalpinx or supporting pelvic ligaments, tubal spasm or abrupt changes in intra-abdominal pressure due to vomiting or coughing have all been proposed as mechanisms which may predispose the normal ovary to torsion [6,16,18].

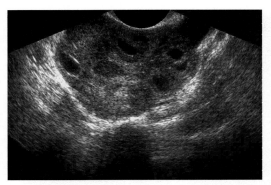

Fig. 5. This 34 year old woman presented with acute pelvic pain. The ovary is enlarged with distortion of the normal architecture. Note several scattered cystic areas, some with thick walls, and irregular areas of increased echogenicity consistent with hemorrhage.

US findings of ovarian torsion

The gray scale, color and Doppler US findings of adnexal torsion are quite variable and are likely dependent upon the duration of symptoms, degree or torsion, whether the torsion is intermittent,

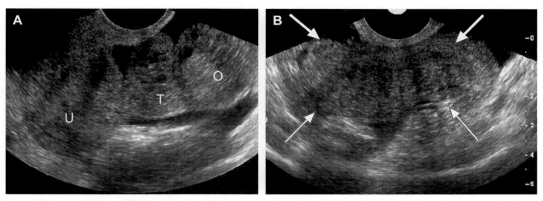

Fig. 7. (A) Note thickened fallopian tube (T) between the uterus (U) and Ovary (O) in a patient with adnexal torsion. *(B)* Longitudinal endovaginal US image through elongated thickened fallopian tube *(arrows)*.

whether or not an ipsilateral ovarian mass is present, and whether the fallopian tube is twisted along with the ovary.

The ovary is enlarged and tender on examination in virtually all cases of ovarian torsion. The enlarged ovary is often abnormal in location, midline and superior to the uterus (see Fig. 1). An enlarged ovary with prominent heterogeneous central stroma and small peripheral follicles has been described as the "classic" gray scale US appearance of ovarian torsion (Figs. 1B and 2) [19–22]. Within the central stroma, echogenic components likely reflect hemorrhage and hypoechoic areas are believed to represent interstitial edema. While this pattern is

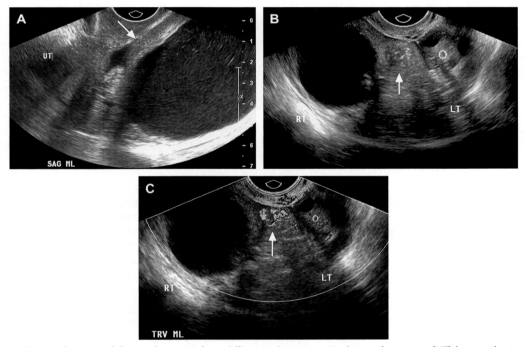

Fig. 8. Gray scale image *(A)* reveals a complex midline cystic mass posterior to the uterus (UT) in a patient who presented with 3 days of intermittent mild pelvic pain. Note internal echoes in the cystic component of the mass consistent with hemorrhage and asymmetric thickening of the cyst wall *(arrow)* which is thickest adjacent to the uterus. *(B)* Note "whirlpool" or target sign *(arrow)* between cyst and left ovary (O) representing the twisted fallopian tube on transverse gray scale image. *(C)* Color Doppler image reveals blood vessels *(arrow)* in this area. Left ovary (O). At surgery, a chronically infarcted ovary virtually replaced by a blood filled sac without recognizable ovarian parenchyma was observed.

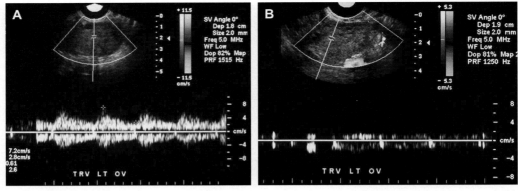

Fig. 9. This 28 year old woman presented with acute onset of LLQ pain. Doppler interrogation revealed both arterial (*A*) and venous flow (*B*) in the ovary although complete torsion was found at surgery.

highly suggestive of ovarian torsion, several authors report that it is inconsistently seen [12,20–23]. This pattern may be more common in early, incomplete or intermittent torsion which may nonetheless cause obstruction of lymphatic and venous drainage resulting in an increase in hydrostatic capillary pressure and ovarian edema [19]. Otherwise, the ovary that has undergone torsion may appear quite complex (Figs. 3–5). An underlying mass such as a dermoid cyst or serous/hemorrhagic cyst, may be observed (Fig. 6). A cystic adnexal mass may have a smoothly or eccentrically thickened wall. Thickening of the fallopian tube may be visualized as an adjacent heterogenous fusiform or tubular structure between the adnexal mass and the uterus (Fig. 7). On cross section, the enlarged tube may have a laminated or "target-like" appearance with alternating hypoechoic and echogenic bands (Fig. 8A). The hypoechoic bands are believed to represent the twisted vessels in the adnexal pedicle and can best be appreciated on color Doppler imaging (Fig. 8B) unless the vessels are thrombosed. This has been described as the whirlpool sign by Vijayaraghavan [24] (234 and is best observed by rotating the probe "to and fro" perpendicular to the longitudinal plane of the thickened tube. Lee and

colleagues [20] observed the twisted vascular pedicle on US in 87% of cases in their series. It is reportedly harder to detect the twisted pedicle if there is less than a 360° twist or if the pedicle is small. Tortuous adnexal vessels can possibly cause false positive examinations in patients with pelvic inflammatory disease, hemorrhagic cysts or endometriosis [23]. However, not all authors report detecting the enlarged fallopian tube or twisted vascular pedicle with such frequency on US examination [10,12,25].

The role of Doppler ultrasound in diagnosing ovarian or adnexal torsion remains controversial and findings are quite variable in all reported series. Certainly color Doppler plays an important role in identifying the whirlpool sign as described above, and absence of Doppler detected blood flow in a painful, morphologically abnormal ovary is highly suspicious of ovarian torsion/infarction. However, normal arterial and venous pulse Doppler waveforms can occasionally be detected in ovaries with surgically confirmed torsion (Fig. 9) [3,10–12]. Hence, a normal ovarian Doppler examination does not exclude ovarian torsion (Fig. 10). Explanations for preservation of Doppler detected ovarian blood flow include the dual arterial supply

Fig. 10. In this patient with acute onset of right lower quadrant pain and surgically proven ovarian torsion, gray scale images (*A,B*) reveal the classic appearance of ovarian torsion: prominent central stoma, peripheral cysts and increased size of the right ovary in comparison to the left ovary seen in image (*C*). (*D*) Doppler interrogation reveals a normal arterial waveform on the right. (*E*) T$_2$ weighted sagittal (*E*) and axial (*F*) MR images demonstrate an enlarged right ovary midline and superior to the uterus with increased signal intensity of the central ovarian stroma on the right consistent with edema and peripherally displaced follicles. Note thickened fallopian tube between uterus and right ovary (*arrow in F*). There is a small amount of ascites. (*G*) Axial contrast enhanced T1 weighted MR image reveals similar findings. The right ovary does not enhance while the left ovarian parenchyma enhances normally. Note thickened fallopian tube between uterus and right ovary (*arrow*) and minimal wall enhancement of the follicular walls on the right which is commonly seen on MRI in patients with ovarian torsion. (*H*) 3 months post surgical untwisting of the right ovary, follow up US demonstrates that the right ovary is decreased in size with a normal appearance of the ovarian parenchyma.

to the ovary from both the ovarian and uterine arteries, partial torsion resulting in obstruction to lymphatic and venous drainage before arterial occlusion occurs, and intermittent torsion such that the US examination is performed during a period of spontaneous detorsion when blood flow has been temporarily restored. It is postulated that as the ovarian vascular pedicle twists, lymphatic drainage is first obstructed resulting in stromal edema and swelling. Next, venous outflow is compromised

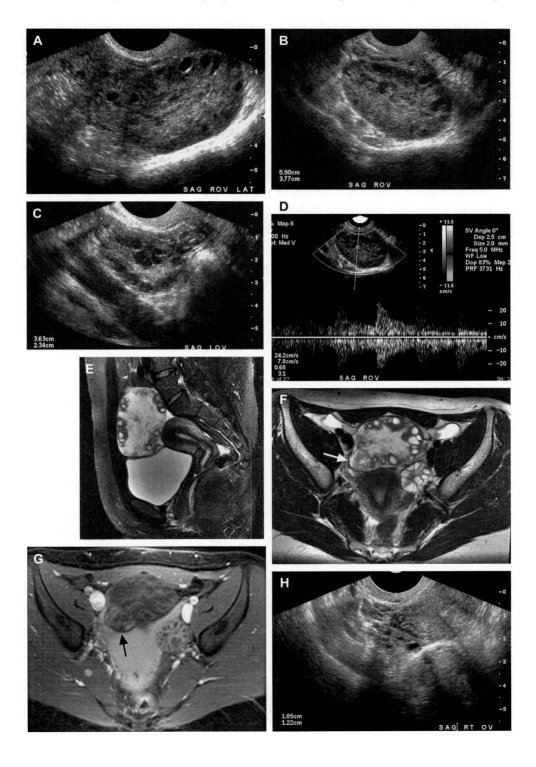

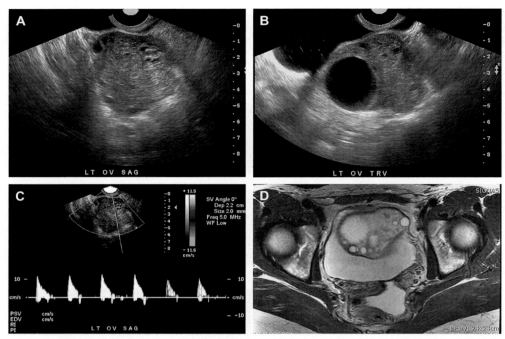

Fig. 11. Gray scale images (*A,B*) in this patient presenting with LLQ pain reveal a rounded amorphous left ovary with peripheral follicles and a dominant cyst. Decreased diastolic flow is noted on pulse Doppler interrogation (*C*) although peak systolic velocity is normal. (*D*) Axial T$_2$ weighted MR image demonstrates classic features of ovarian torsion: an enlarged round ovary in the midline demonstrating increased signal intensity of the central stroma and peripheral follicles.

resulting in decreased venous flow or venous thrombosis. Decreased diastolic and/or peak systolic arterial flow then occurs secondary to increased peripheral vascular resistance resulting from increased interstitial pressure from transudation of fluid from increased hydrostatic pressure (Fig. 11), and finally, arterial flow will cease (see Fig. 2). Hence, complete absence of flow appears to be a late finding of ovarian torsion and an insensitive but highly specific criterion [3,12].

There are several important technical factors which must be considered in order to optimize the Doppler US exam and avoid false positive or false negative examinations. The ovary should be interrogated in multiple imaging planes and venous as well as arterial flow should always be assessed. Machine settings should optimize detection of low velocity, slow flow. The pulse repetition frequency (PRF), color velocity scale, and wall filter should be set low. The color gain should be set as high as possible before the image is degraded by color flash motion artifact and the gray scale/color priority setting should be optimized [12,26–28]. Occasionally, the ovary is so deep in the pelvis that blood flow cannot be detected on transvaginal Doppler ultrasound interrogation despite optimization of machine settings. In some cases using

a transabdominal approach with a lower frequency transducer may be helpful. However, one should always be cautious in making the presumptive diagnosis of ovarian torsion in a morphologically normal ovary even if no blood flow is detected on Doppler US examination. Conversely, if the ovary looks suspicious morphologically but blood flow appears normal, torsion should still be considered.

It is more difficult to diagnose ovarian torsion in the presence of an underlying ipsilateral ovarian mass [10] or when only the fallopian tube alone is torqued (Fig. 12). In a patient with a hemorrhagic or leaking ovarian cyst, it can be incorrectly assumed that the underlying pathology is the cause of the patient's acute pelvic pain and the associated ovarian torsion may be overlooked (see Fig. 6; Fig. 13). In patients with large cystic teratomas it may be difficult to see the adjacent ovary and fallopian tube, either because of displacement out of the field of view or shadowing/attenuation from calcifications or fat. In addition, blood flow is rarely observed on Doppler US examination of an asymptomatic cystic teratoma. However, in a patient with acute pain and an ovarian cystic teratoma, adnexal torsion or rupture of the cystic teratoma should be suspected (Fig. 14) even in the absence of discrete findings if the adjacent ovary is not

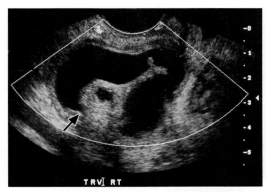

Fig. 12. Torsed Fallopian Tube. This patient presented with acute pelvic pain. Color Doppler image reveals an avascular complex right adnexal mass containing a dilated fallopian tube. Note "beak-like" configuration (*arrow*) where the tube is twisted around the ovary. At surgery only the dilated fallopian tube was torsed.

visualized. It is also difficult to make the diagnosis of ovarian torsion in a patient with enlarged hyperstimulated ovaries as the ovarian architecture is distorted by the presence of the numerous follicles in addition to the common baseline findings of edema and hemorrhage within the ovarian stroma. With so many follicles present, peripheral displacement of the follicles is difficult to detect. In addition, hyperstimulated ovaries may be asymmetrically enlarged and blood flow is typically increased which could potentially limit the sensitivity of the Doppler US examination (Fig. 15). Nonetheless, asymmetry in size, blood flow, and tenderness on either physical or US examination can be clues to the diagnosis.

The role of Doppler US in differentiating the viable from non viable ovary is also controversial.

Complete absence of flow in a technically adequate exam suggests ovarian infarction. Lee and colleagues [23] and Vijayaraghavan [24] have suggested that absence of flow in the twisted tube or vascular pedicle suggests that the ovary is non-viable, and Fleischer and colleagues [28] found absent central flow to be a worrisome finding. Conversely, small ovarian size [28], normal venous ovarian flow [28] and flow in the twisted pedicle [23,24] have been reported to be associated with ovarian viability. However, experience is limited and the available data is somewhat conflicting. Thus, the role of US in determining viability of the torsed ovary requires further evaluation.

CT appearance of ovarian torsion

US remains the first line imaging modality of choice for evaluation of patients with suspected gynecologic pathology and has been shown to be more accurate and sensitive than either CT or MRI for diagnosing adnexal torsion [10]. However, CT is frequently the first imaging study obtained in women with non-specific pelvic pain. Thus, since patients with adnexal torsion may present with mild or intermittent lower quadrant pain over several days or even months, one may first image a patient with ovarian torsion on CT. Hence, the radiologist should be familiar with the CT findings of ovarian torsion.

The most common imaging finding of adnexal torsion on CT is the presence of an adnexal mass. However, this is an extremely non-specific finding. The ovary may be enlarged and displaced into the midline either anteriorly or in the cul de sac (Fig. 16) [10]. Smooth, eccentric thickening (>3 mm) of the wall of a cystic adnexal mass and an adjacent

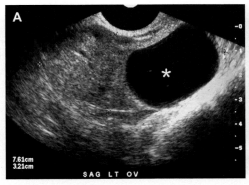

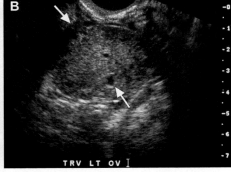

Fig. 13. This 34 year old woman presented with acute onset of LLQ pain. (*A*) Initial US revealed an enlarged left ovary (calipers) with a large anechoic ovarian cyst (*) and a small amount of free fluid (not shown). Pain was initially interpreted as due to leakage from the ovarian cyst. However, note rounded configuration of the ovary (*B*) with loss of architectural detail and peripherally displaced follicles (*arrows*) which is suggestive of torsion. When the patient returned 2 days later with persistent pain, adnexal torsion with a necrotic ovary was found at surgery.

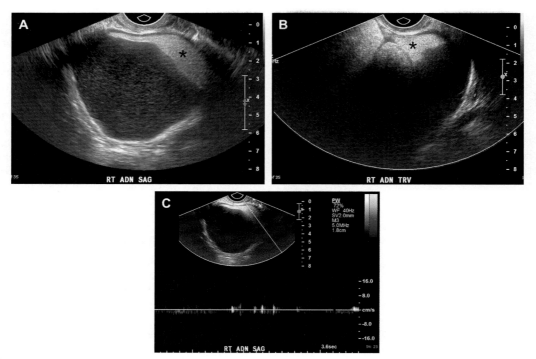

Fig. 14. This patient with a known ovarian dermoid cyst presented with acute RLQ pain. (*A,B*) A large right dermoid cyst is noted. Note anterior echogenic component (*) representing fat with posterior attenuation (*B*). The left ovary was not identified. Neither color Doppler (*B*) nor pulse Doppler (*C*) interrogation reveal blood flow. However, lack of blood flow is not a specific finding of torsion in dermoid cysts as Doppler interrogation rarely demonstrates blood flow in asymptomatic dermoids. Nonetheless torsion must be considered due to the clinical presentation despite the lack of specific US findings. This dermoid had undergone complete torsion at surgery.

enlarged fallopian tube are considered the most specific findings of ovarian torsion [29–31]. However, smooth circumferential thickening of the wall of a cyst >10 mm without evidence of tumor-like nodularity or irregularity is also a suspicious finding

[29,30]. Adjacent hematoma may be noted (Fig. 17). Thickened fallopian tubes most commonly appear on CT as an amorphous or tubular solid mass located between the adnexal mass and ovary. The thickened fallopian tube may be draped

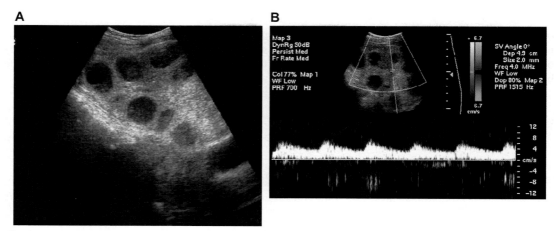

Fig. 15. Ovarian torsion in a pregnant patient with ovarian hyperstimulation syndrome. (*A*) Note markedly enlarged ovary with numerous cysts. (*B*) Color Doppler imaging reveals diminished flow, but spectral Doppler interrogation demonstrates central arterial flow. The ovarian pedicle was twisted three full rotations at surgery.

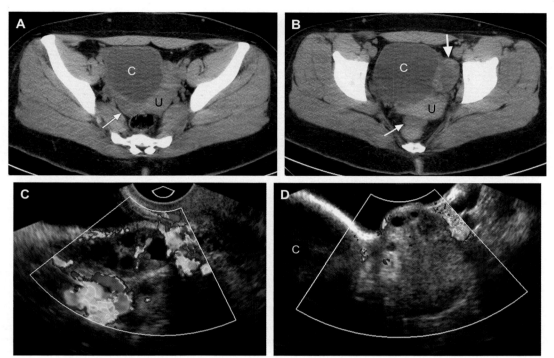

Fig. 16. (*A*) CT scan without intravenous contrast demonstrates a normal sized right ovary (*arrow*). The uterus (U) is mildly deviated to the left of midline. The large low-density mass (C), found to be a left paraovarian cyst at surgery, is located anterior to the uterus secondary to torsion. The abnormal location of the mass and the enlarged left ovary anterior to the uterus is suggestive of adnexal torsion; abnormal location of the ovary maybe more readily appreciated on CT and MRI in comparison to ultrasound. (*B*) CT scan without intravenous contrast caudal to (*A*) demonstrates the low-density mass (C) and an enlarged left ovary (*large arrow*), both located anterior to the uterus (U). There is a small amount of fluid in the cul de sac (*small arrow*). (*C*) Transvaginal sonogram with color Doppler demonstrates normal right ovary. (*D*) Transvaginal sonogram with color Doppler shows enlarged left ovary with minimal, if any, vascular flow. A few small peripheral follicles are identified. Note the increased echogenicity of this torsed left ovary. Only a small portion of the left paraovarian cyst is seen on this image (C).

partially over the mass or demonstrate a "beak-like" protrusion [10,29,30]. These features may be more easily depicted on coronal or sagittal reconstructions. Central high attenuation suggests hemorrhage which is more commonly present if infarction has occurred [10,30]. If intravenous (IV) contrast has been administered, the mass may have a whirled or "target-like" appearance representing the twisted vascular pedicle [29]. However, a thickened fallopian tube may occasionally be difficult to differentiate from unopacified loops of bowel [30]. Rha and colleagues [28] observed tubal thickening in 84% and smooth thickening of the wall of a cystic mass in 76% of their 25 patients with surgically proven adnexal torsion, all of whom had an underlying adnexal mass. In this series, eccentric wall thickening was twice as common as concentric thickening and occurred adjacent to the thickened fallopian tube.

Convergence of engorged blood vessels and the presence of dilated but, straight blood vessels running over the mass have also been described as an uncommon but specific finding of adnexal torsion on CT [31], likely representing congested and tethered adnexal veins. Hence, if ovarian torsion is suspected, contrast enhanced imaging should be timed to depict arterial flow in the twisted pedicle as well as delayed venous congestion. Differentiation of engorged veins due to torsion or pelvic venous congestion from other inflammatory processes may be difficult [30].

Lack of contrast enhancement in an adnexal mass is suggestive of torsion [29,31] although this is a non-specific finding as cystic adnexal structures do not normally enhance on CT except for their walls. In addition, cyst wall enhancement may be observed in patients with adnexal torsion if the torsion is intermittent or incomplete. Rha and colleagues [29] postulate if the wall of an adnexal cystic structure enhances but internal septations do not, torsion should be considered. However,

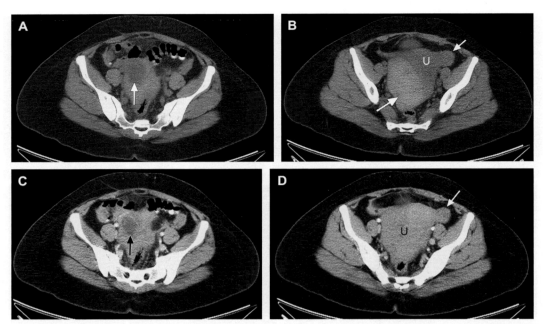

Fig. 17. (*A*) CT scan at the level of the mid pelvis before administration of IV contrast demonstrates a low density mass in the right adnexal region (*arrow*) surrounded by high density hematoma. (*B*) CT scan caudal to (*A*) before IV contrast shows high density hematoma (*large arrow*) to the right of the uterus (U) and extending into the cul de sac (*large arrow*). Note that the left ovary (*small arrow*) is of soft tissue density similar to the uterus (U). (*C*) CT scan after IV contrast shows non-enhancement of the right adnexal mass (*arrow*), indicating necrosis of the torsed right ovary, surrounded by hematoma. (*D*) CT scan caudal to (*C*) after IV contrast shows normal enhancement of the uterus (U) and left ovary (*arrow*). The uterus is displaced slightly to the left by the right pelvic hematoma which is seen better on the non-contrast images (*A,B*).

fibrin strands within a hemorrhagic cyst also will not enhance on CT. Other less commonly reported and less specific findings of ovarian torsion on CT include ascites [10,29–31], deviation of the uterus to the affected side (see **Fig. 16**) [10,29,30], and hazy stranding from inflammation or hemorrhage in the surrounding pelvic fat (**Fig. 16**) [10,30,31].

An infarcted ovary must be surgically removed as it is a potential nidus for infection. However, a viable torsed ovary can be safely untwisted and left in situ, thereby preserving ovarian function. Since ovarian viability cannot always be determined on physical inspection at the time of surgery, it would be useful if imaging features could differentiate an infarcted from a viable torsed ovary. The literature on CT diagnosis of ovarian infarction versus viability is limited. However, it seems likely that an ovary which demonstrates no IV contrast enhancement is likely infarcted (see **Fig. 17**) [10]. In addition, the "beak-like" configuration of the thickened fallopian tube, adjacent distended and straightened blood vessels, as well as, converging blood vessels have been reported by Kimura and colleagues [30] as signs of ovarian infarction. However, their sample size was small. Adjacent hematoma and stranding

with in the pelvic fat have also been described as a findings associated with ovarian infarction (see **Fig. 17**) [10]. Yashiro and colleagues [32] reported the finding of air within an ovarian tumor or in adjacent veins to be suggestive of infarction. Rha and colleagues [29] reported lack of enhancement of central septations and hemorrhage within the fallopian tube to be associated with ovarian infarction. However, in their series of 25 patients, the only statistically significant difference between patients with and without hemorrhagic ovarian infarction was the presence of eccentric cyst wall thickening >10 mm (*P*<.05) [29].

MR appearance of ovarian torsion

MRI is likely more accurate than CT in diagnosing ovarian/adnexal torsion and in differentiating an infarcted from a viable torsed ovary due to the multiplanar imaging capability and increased soft tissue resolution of MRI. However, since it is often difficult to obtain an MRI emergently, MRI is rarely obtained as an initial, immediate diagnostic study in patients presenting acutely with pelvic pain. Thus, MRI is most effectively ultilized for evaluation of

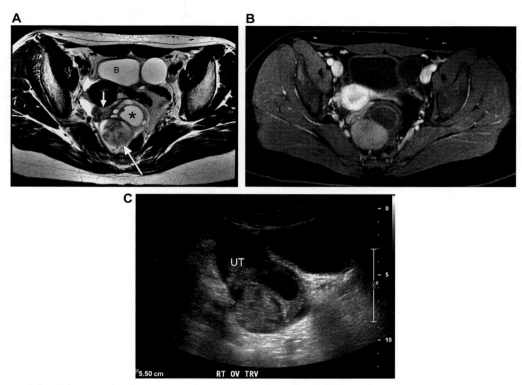

Fig. 18. (A) Axial T$_2$ weighted MR image demonstrates the twisted thickened ovarian pedicle or fallopian tube (*short arrow*) coursing between the uterus and an enlarged right ovary which contains both a hemorrhagic (*long arrow*) and serous cyst (*). The residual ovarian tissue demonstrates peripherally displaced follicles and increased signal intensity in the ovarian stroma. A simple cyst on the left ovary is noted lateral to the bladder (*B*). There is no enhancement of the ovarian parenchyma on the right although the twisted fallopian tube minimally enhances on the post contrast T$_1$ weighted axial image (*B*) in this 14 year old girl who presented with 2 days of pelvic pain due to ovarian torsion. Minimal enhancement of the wall of the right ovarian serous cyst is noted. (*C*) A transverse gray scale image from the initial US examination demonstrates an enlarged ovary with a hemorrhagic cyst and peripheral follicles. Note that the right ovary is abnormally located in the left side of the pelvis. Uterus (UT). Arterial flow to the right ovary was normal on Doppler interrogation (not shown). (*Courtesy of Dr. T. Robin Goodman, MD, New Haven, CT.*)

patients with pelvic pain or an adnexal mass in whom the initial US or CT examination is non-diagnostic or in whom the clinical presentation is atypical for ovarian torsion. Hence, the MR findings of ovarian/adnexal torsion described below apply primarily to subacute or chronic cases.

In cases of suspected ovarian torsion, the MR imaging protocol should consist of T1 weighted images with and without fat suppression as well as T2 weighted sequences in axial and sagittal planes with additional coronal views as necessary. These sequences will help identify hemorrhage as well as fat within the adnexa. The presence of fat within an adnexal mass is diagnostic of a cystic teratoma, the most common ovarian neoplasm found in torsed ovaries. Pre and post IV gadolinium T1 weighted fat suppressed images ($\pm$ subtraction techniques) should also be obtained to assess for

contrast enhancement in the ovarian stroma, solid components of any underlying mass, cyst walls, and the fallopian tube.

Imaging findings of ovarian torsion on MRI are similar to what has been previously described for CT: namely a thick, edematous adjacent tube or pedicle (see Fig. 10; Fig. 18) [10,25,29,31,33–35], engorged vessels adjacent to the tumor [31,33,35] or draped around the tumor [33], enlarged ovary [25,34] and smooth, often eccentric, thickening of the wall of an ipsilateral ovarian cyst [29]. Adnexal hematoma [10,36] complex adnexal masses with heterogeneous enhancement [10,37,38] and lack of contrast enhancement of an adnexal mass [31] have also been described on MR in patients with adnexal torsion. Engorged blood vessels and the tubular nature of the thickened fallopian tube coursing between the ovarian mass and uterus with a "beak-like" or "pinched-off" appearance at the site of torsion are more easily detected on MR than CT due to it's multiplanar capability and soft tissue resolution which enhances detection of blood vessels. Abnormal midline location of an enlarged ovary and infiltration of the pelvic fat have also been described on MR as findings suggestive of ovarian torsion (see Figs. 10 and 18) [10].

However, the most specific MR appearance of ovarian torsion is quite similar to the "classic" US appearance of ovarian torsion. The ovary is markedly enlarged with numerous small peripheral follicles and the central ovarian stroma demonstrates bright (similar to water) signal intensity on T2 weighted images due to edema from vascular congestion and/or lymphatic obstruction (see Fig. 10) [25,34–38]. Several authors speculate that when the underlying ovarian architecture is thus preserved and some enhancement is seen, especially in the walls of the follicles, that the ovary remains viable and can be successfully detorsed (see Fig. 10) [25,36]. Increased signal intensity on T1 weighted images suggests hemorrhage and complete lack of contrast enhancement of the ovary suggests infarction (see Fig. 18) [25,29,34].

Summary

The most common presentation of adnexal torsion, which usually involves both the ovary and fallopian tube, is acute lower abdominal or pelvic pain along with nausea and vomiting. However, atypical presentations, including mild or intermittent symptoms over several days and associated leukocytosis, may mimic other gynecologic conditions such as hemorrhagic/ruptured ovarian cysts, ectopic pregnancy or pelvic inflammatory disease and even gastrointestinal or renal pathology resulting in delayed diagnosis. Transvaginal sonography with Doppler interrogation remains the most accurate and effective imaging modality for the diagnosis of adnexal torsion [10]. However, it is important to be familiar with the CT findings of adnexal torsion as CT may be the first imaging study performed in the setting of non-specific signs and symptoms. Limited experience indicates that MRI with or without intravenous contrast is useful in cases where the sonographic and/or CT findings are equivocal, especially in the pregnant patient or in patients with an underlying adnexal mass. While most cases of adnexal torsion occur in women of reproductive age, the possibility of adnexal torsion should not be ignored in children and post-menopausal women. Common risk factors include ipsilateral adnexal mass, prior pelvic surgery, pregnancy, and ovarian hyperstimulation syndrome.

References

[1] Hibbard LT. Adnexal torsion. Am J Obstet Gynecol 1985;152:456–61.

[2] Burnett LS. Gynecologic causes of the acute abdomen. Surg Clin North Am 1988;68:385–98.

[3] Pena JE, Ufberg D, Cooney N, et al. Usefulness of Doppler sonography in the diagnosis of ovarian torsion. Fertil Steril 2000;73:1047–50.

[4] Nichols DH, Julian PJ. Torsion of the adnexa. Clin Obstet Gynecol 1985;28:375–80.

[5] Wagaman R, Williams RS. Conservative therapy for adnexal torsion—a case report. J Reprod Med 1990;35:833–4.

[6] Breech LL, Adams Hillard PJ. Adnexal torsion in pediatric and adolescent girls. Curr Opin Obstet Gynecol 2005;17:483–9.

[7] Bider D, Mashiach S, Dulitzky M, et al. Clinical, surgical and pathologic findings of adnexal torsion in pregnant and nonpregnant women. Surg Gynecol Obstet 1991;173:363–6.

[8] Houry D, Abbott JT. Ovarian torsion: a fifteen-year review. Ann Emerg Med 2001;38(2): 156–9.

[9] Lee RA, Welch JS. Torsion of the uterine adnexa. Am J Obstet Gynecol 1967;97:974–7.

[10] Chiou SE, Lev-Toaff AS, Masuda E, et al. Adnexal torsion: new clinical and imaging observations by sonography, computed tomography, and magnetic resonance imaging. J Ultrasound Med 2007;26:1289–301.

[11] Rosado WM, Trambert MA, Gosink BB, et al. Adnexal torsion: diagnosis using doppler sonography. AJR Am J Roentgenol 1992;159:1251–3.

[12] Albayram F, Hamper UM. Ovarian and adnexal torsion. J Ultrasound Med 2001;20:1083–9.

[13] Desai SK, Allahbadia GN, Dalal AK. Ovarian torsion: diagnosis by color Doppler ultrasonography. Obstet Gynecol 1994;84:699–701.

[14] Ignacio EA, Hill MC. Ultrasound of the acute female pelvis. Ultrasound Q 2003;19(2):86–98.

[15] Stark JE, Siegel MJ. Ovarian torsion in prepubertal and pubertal girls: sonographic findings. AJR Am J Roentgenol 1994;163:1479–82.

[16] Kokoska ER, Keller MS, Weber TR, et al. Acute ovarian torsion in children. Am J Surg 2000;180:462–5.

[17] Warner BW, Kuhn JC, Barr LL. Conservative management of large ovarian cysts in children: the value of serial pelvic ultrasonography. Surgery 1992;112:749–55.

[18] Mordehai J, Mares AJ, Barki Y, et al. Torsion of uterine adnexa in neonates and children: a report of 20 cases. J Pediatr Surg 1991;26:1195–9.

[19] Warner MA, Fleischer AC, Edell SL, et al. Uterine adnexal torsion: sonographic findings. Radiology 1985;154:773–5.

[20] Graif M, Itzchak Y. Sonographic evaluation of ovarian torsion in childhood and adolescence. AJR Am J Roentgenol 1988;150:647–9.

[21] Graif M, Shalev J, Strauss S, et al. Torsion of the ovary: sonographic features. AJR Am J Roentgenol 1984;143:1331–4.

[22] Helvie MA, Silver TM. Ovarian torsion: sonographic evaluation. J Clin Ultrasound 1989;17: 327–32.

[23] Lee EJ, Kwon HC, Joo HJ, et al. Diagnosis of ovarian torsion with color doppler sonography: depiction of twisted vascular pedicle. J Ultrasound Med 1998;17:83–9.

[24] Vijayaraghavan SB. Sonographic whirlpool sign in ovarian torsion. J Ultrasound Med 2004;23: 1643–9.

[25] Ghossain MA, Hachem K, Buy JN, et al. Adnexal torsion: magnetic resonance findings in the viable adnexa with emphasis on stromal ovarian appearance. J Magn Reson Imaging 2004;20: 451–62.

[26] Pellerito JS, Troiano RN, Quedens-Case C, et al. Common pitfalls of endovaginal color doppler flow imaging. Radiographics 1995;15:37–47.

[27] Lambert M, Villa M. Gynecologic ultrasound in emergency medicine. Emerg Med Clin North Am 2004;22:683–96.

[28] Fleischer AC, Stein SM, Cullinan JA, et al. Color Doppler sonography of adnexal torsion. J Ultrasound Med 1995;14:523–8.

[29] Rha SE, Byun JY, Jung SE, et al. CT and MR imaging features of adnexal torsion. Radiographics 2002;22:283–94.

[30] Kim YH, Cho KS, Ha HK, et al. CT features of torsion of benign cystic teratoma of the ovary. J Comput Assist Tomogr 1999;23(6): 923–8.

[31] Kimura I, Togashi K, Kawakami S, et al. Ovarian torsion: CT and MR imaging appearances. Radiology 1994;190:337–41.

[32] Yasuhiro K, Toshio F, Sakne F, et al. Intravascular gas within an ovarian tumor: a CT sign of ovarian torsion. J Comput Assist Tomogr 1996;20: 154–6.

[33] VanKerkhove F, Cannie M, Op de Beeck K, et al. Ovarian torsion in a premenarchal girl: MRI findings. Abdom Imaging 2007;32:424–7.

[34] Tamia K, Koyama T, Saga T, et al. MR features of physiologic and benign conditions of the ovary. Eur Radiol 2006;16:2700–11.

[35] Nishino M, Hayakawa K, Iwasaku K, et al. Magnetic resonance imaging findings in gynecologic emergencies. J Comput Assist Tomogr 2003;27: 564–70.

[36] Haque TL, Togashi K, Kobayashi H, et al. Adnexal torsion: MR imaging findings of viable ovary. Eur Radiol 2000;10:1954–7.

[37] Kramer LA, Lalani T, Kawashima A. Massive edema of the ovary: high resolution MR findings using a phased-array pelvic coil. J Magn Reson Imaging 1997;7:758–60.

[38] Lee AR, Kim KH, Lee BH, et al. Massive edema of the ovary: imaging findings. AJR Am J Roentgenol 1993;161:343–4.

ULTRASOUND CLINICS

Ultrasound Clin 2 (2007) 327–332

Index

Note: Page numbers of article titles are in **boldface** type.

1556-858X/07/$ – see front matter © 2007 Elsevier Inc. All rights reserved.   doi:10.1016/S1556-858X(07)00089-8
ultrasound.theclinics.com